DEPARTMENT OF HEALTH AND SOCIAL SERVICES

ADULT DENTAL HEALTH SURVEY NORTHERN IRELAND 1979

A survey conducted by the Department of
Health and Social Services in collaboration with the
Social Research Division of the Central Economic Service

J. R. Rhodes and
T. H. Haire

BELFAST
HER MAJESTY'S STATIONERY OFFICE

Acknowledgements

Many people made a contribution to the Survey. Due to the limitations of space it would be impossible to thank every person who provided help in one form or another but certain individuals and certain bodies must be mentioned.

The Survey was made as similar as possible to other Adult Dental Health Surveys which have taken place within the United Kingdom. This was done in order to make the results of the Northern Ireland Survey comparable with the results of the other surveys. Demands were thus made on the expertise and time of the staff who had planned and organised the 1978 Survey of Adult Dental Health in the United Kingdom. We would like to express appreciation for the help provided by Jean Todd and Alison Walker of the Office of Population Censuses and Surveys and for similar help provided by the staff of Birmingham Dental School, in particular Dr. R. J. Anderson. Dr. Roger Anderson provided invaluable advice on the calibration exercises and provided a considerable quantity of teaching material. He also took a personal interest in the arrangements for the training of the dental examiners and scrutinised the training courses prepared by the Northern Ireland tutors. Mr. Peter Hull of Manchester University Dental School who had participated in the training exercises for the UK Survey also helped with the periodontal component of the training courses.

Special thanks are due to Mr. Jeremy Harbison, Head of the Social Research Division of the Central Economic Service for his supervision of the planning and organisation of the Survey and for his examination of and comments on the draft of this report. Our thanks go also to Mr. Ivan Houston and his staff who checked and coded the questionnaires and to Mr. Richard Pearce.

Models, appliances and other teaching materials were supplied by Mr. G. A. S. Blair and Mr. Andrew Richardson of the School of Dentistry, Queen's University of Belfast, by Messrs. R. Y. Black and H. G. McKinley and by Mrs. P. D. Wilson, who was also a training course tutor. We are very grateful for their help.

We would like to thank the volunteer examinees from the staff of the Department of Health and Social Services, from the Social Research Division and from the Staffs Council who kindly consented to act as "guinea-pigs" during the dental examination practice sessions. We would also like to thank Mr. Trevor Mitchell of the Department of Health and Social Services for his contributions to the survey and the training sessions.

Lastly we would like to express our thanks to the members of the public who provided information by answering questions at interview and by submitting to a dental examination. They were kind enough to open their homes to the interviewers and examiners. Without their co-operation, the survey would have been impossible.

NOTE: In order to make comparison as easy as possible this report has been presented in a similar manner to those of the England and Wales[1] and Scotland[2] surveys. Acknowledgement is therefore due to the writers of these reports.

1. Adult Dental Health in England and Wales in 1968 by P. G. Gray, J. E. Todd, G. L. Slack and J. S. Bulman. HMSO 1970.
2. Adult Dental Health in Scotland 1972 by J. E. Todd and A. Whitworth. HMSO 1974.

Contents

1. Introduction

Early in 1979 the Department of Health and Social Services asked the Social Research Division of the Central Economic Service of the Department of Finance to carry out a survey of adult dental health. No such survey had previously been carried out in Northern Ireland. Although Northern Ireland had been included in the United Kingdom Adult Dental Health Survey of 1978 the Northern Ireland sample was selected on a United Kingdom population basis and was thus too small to permit analysis of the results for Northern Ireland alone.

In order to ensure that the results of the Northern Ireland survey were compatible with the results of the United Kingdom Survey of 1978, the same interview schedules and dental record charts were used and the tutors for the Northern Ireland calibration courses had taken part in the United Kingdom survey. The teaching material was similar to that used in the 1978 survey and where possible the same material was used. Dr. R. J. Anderson of Birmingham University very kindly advised on the content and material used in the calibration course to ensure that the criteria were the same as in the United Kingdom survey.

1.1 Outline of the Survey

Social Research Division selected a random sample of adults from the Electoral Register. Experienced social research interviewers were employed by the Division to collect information for the survey. Each interviewer attended a training seminar which was designed to accustom the interviewer to the dental schedules. Each interviewer was also trained in the recording of dental conditions.

The persons selected in the sample were approached by the interviewers and asked if they would consent to take part in the survey. Those consenting were interviewed. On completion of the interview, dentate persons were asked to co-operate further by permitting a dental examination to be carried out in the home. If consent was given, the interviewer returned at a suitable time with a dentist who carried out the examination. The interviewer acted as recorder during the dental examination.

1.2 The Sample

The survey sample was made up of persons over 16 years of age resident in private homes. Persons resident in institutions were excluded from the sample because of the sampling and interview difficulties. A similar exclusion was made in the United Kingdom Adult Dental Health Survey.

Because of the small size of Northern Ireland a larger sample had to be selected than was warranted by the proportion of the United Kingdom population resident in Northern Ireland. In order to provide meaningful results the sample population had to be increased as had been done for Scotland and Wales in the 1978 survey. While the inclusion of the Northern Ireland results in their correct proportion allowed the presentation of data on a UK basis, a much larger sample was necessary for the purposes of analysis and comparison.

For this reason the sample of 160 persons used in the UK survey was replaced by a larger sample from 1,517 addresses. The electoral register was used as a basis for the selection of both samples. Persons selected for the Northern Ireland sample of the UK survey were not excluded from the sample. Further details of the sample are given in Table 1.1. and Appendix 1.

TABLE 1.1

	N.I.	%	U.K.	%
(a) Sample of addresses				
Number of addresses selected	1,517		7,266	
Withdrawn (institutions empty, or demolished)	51		113	
			7,153	
No one available for interview at address	91		878	
Actual sample of available addresses	1,375		6,275	
(b) Co-operation achieved for interview		%		%
Interview obtained	1,176	86	5,967	89
Refusal	35	2	529	8
Non-contact (including—out all calls, away each survey period) . .	164	12	183	3
Total people selected from addresses: 1,375 (N.I.); 6,275 (U.K.) . .	1,375	100	6,679	100
(c) Co-operation obtained for dental examination		%		%
Dental examination obtained	592	76	3,495	86
Refusal at end of interview	77	10	398	10
Refusal at second call	83	10	96	2
Non-contact at second call	31	4	93	2
Persons interviewed who had some natural teeth	783	100	4,082	100

1.3 The Examiners

The survey consisted of two elements, the interview and the dental examination. The Social Research Division of the Central Economic Service is engaged in many surveys in the course of a year and maintains a field force of interviewers. It does not however have a team of dental examiners.

In the UK Survey community dental officers carried out the examinations with one or two exceptions and for the Northern Ireland survey the community dental service was asked to provide the dental examiners. The staffing structure of the service is variable, some areas are very short of dental staff and there were difficulties in meeting the requirements for dental examinations in some areas. The difficulties were overcome by some dental examiners travelling considerable distances to their allocated examination areas and by the use of former community dental officers to supplement the team of dental examiners. A list of the dental examiners is given in Appendix 2.

The dentists who carried out the dental examinations attended a one week training course before the survey fieldwork began. At the course they learned the criteria and techniques of dental examination and were able to practice the techniques under the observation of dental tutors. The tutors ensured that the criteria matched the criteria of the 1978 UK Adult Dental Health Survey. The tutors had undergone the training exercises of the UK 1978 survey and had participated in it as dental examiners. Calibration and re-calibration exercises were carried out before and after the survey. By examining the same group of patients with the same recorder and comparing the oral conditions noted, it was possible to assess examiner variability.

1.4 The Interviewers

The interviewers used were experienced members of the Social Research Division field force. They attended special briefing sessions in the use of the dental questionnaires. They obtained practice in recording dental conditions on the prescribed survey charts and attended the dental examiners' training course in order to practice recording dental conditions with the examiners with whom they would be working during the survey.

None of them had previous experience of dental surveys.

Both dental examiners and interviewers took part in the training programme and calibration exercises.

Interviews and dental examinations took place in the homes of selected individuals. At the end of the interview the informant was asked to consent to a dental examination if any natural teeth were present in the mouth. Only persons with natural teeth were examined, the edentulous were excluded as in the UK survey. If the informant consented to a dental examination, the interviewer returned to the informant's home a few days later accompanied by the dental examiner. The interviewer recorded the oral conditions identified by the examiner.

The survey information was confidential and the survey staff were pledged to keep it so.

The interviewer was the informant's main contact with the survey. The dental examiner played a subordinate role when home visits were made. This was a deliberate policy in order to prevent the dental examiner being drawn into discussion of the informant's dental health. The examination information was coded so as to preserve the confidentiality of the dental findings.

The dental examination methods and a list of the equipment used is given in Appendix 3.

1.5　The Response

Because there were two elements in the survey, there were two possibilities for non-response. The interviewers attempted to overcome any negative response. The edentulous were told of the importance of everybody participating in the survey whether they had teeth or not. Persons with some natural teeth were encouraged to participate and their doubts or fears allayed as far as possible. The result of the interviewers work can be seen by the fact that a response rate of 86% of interviews was achieved and 76% of dental examinations of persons with some natural teeth. The corresponding figures for the United Kingdom were 89% for interviews and 86% for examinations. (Table 1.1).

Of those persons interviewed 783 had some natural teeth, 76% had a dental examination, 10% refused to have a dental examination when asked at the end of the interview, a further 10% refused on the second call and 4% could not be contacted when the dentist and the interviewer returned. The interval between the interview and the dental examination was deliberately kept brief. In addition each informant was given an appointment so as to know when the interviewer and examiner would call in order to carry out the dental examination. It was hoped that these measures would reduce the number of failures to obtain examinations.

1.6　The Questionnaires

The dental survey data can be divided into two for purposes of analysis, those who have some natural teeth and those who have none. For the convenience of fieldwork however it is more effective to consider the sample under three headings, those who have only natural teeth, those who have lost all their teeth and those who have a combination of their own teeth and dentures.

As in the United Kingdom survey, three different interview questionnaires were used together with a short introductory questionnaire which helped the interviewer to select the appropriate main questionnaire. An extra Northern Ireland questionnaire was introduced at an appropriate time in the interview, irrespective of the type of main questionnaire being used. The 5 questionnaires are shown in Appendix 4.

The questionnaires for persons with only natural teeth and for persons who were edentulous took about thirty five minutes to complete but the questionnaires for persons with partial dentures took about fifty minutes to complete.

1.7　The Dental Examination

The dental examination was concerned with the condition of the teeth, the condition of the soft tissues, the orthodontic status and with details of any dentures present.

Each tooth was recorded as present, missing, unrestorable or crowned. Spaces were recorded as filled by a denture or bridge, remaining as a space or closed by tooth movement. Each surface of each standing tooth was recorded even if the tooth had been crowned or was unrestorable. The codes used for surfaces were sound, decayed, filled or else both decayed and filled. Filling materials were coded as amalgam, gold or a synthetic filling material.

The soft tissue conditions were recorded for six segments of the mouth, left, middle and right, three in the upper and three in the lower jaw. The presence or absence of soft debris, calculus, gingivitis and periodontitis was noted.

The orthodontic status was assessed by assessing the crowding of the teeth for six segments, measuring the overbite (in millimetres), and overjet (in the proportion of the tooth overlapped by the overlapping tooth) and whether the upper front teeth rested in front of the lower lip when the mouth was closed.

Dental anomalies were recorded but only after the examiner and interviewer had left the informant.

Assessment of dentures present included recording a description of the denture and whether it was adversely affecting the oral tissues. As only persons with some natural teeth were eligible for examination, the effects of dentures on the tissues were confined to the effects on natural teeth and their supporting structures.

The criteria for the dental examination will be found in Appendix 5.

1.8　The Examination Technique

The examination in the informant's home was designed to provide an accurate assessment of the informant's oral condition with the minimum inconvenience to the informant. The dental examiner supplied all the materials necessary for the dental examination.* The informant was asked to sit in an upright chair with a high back if one was available. The interviewer who acted as recorder sat nearby within easy earshot of the examiner. The examiner carried a plastic bag with a sponge soaked in a sterilising solution and a towel so that hand cleaning could be done with minimum disturbance. A closed container containing sterilizing solution held probes, mirrors and a rule to measure overjet. The mirrors were No. 4 plane type and the probe tips had been made standard. The examiners were supplied with hand held flexible examination lights† and had been trained in their use prior to the survey examinations.

---

*Dental Examination Kit: Appendix 3.
†Hoyt Laboratories Division of Colgate Palmolive Ltd.

Each examination took about five minutes, but the entry, introductions, laying out equipment, handwashing etc took longer. Most visits lasted less than 15 minutes. Much more time was spent by the dental examiners travelling from one informants home to another than was spent in examinations. In the rural districts quite considerable distances were travelled by both interviewers and examiners.

The examination chart is shown in Appendix 6.

2. The Survey Method

2.1 Coverage

Since the purpose of the survey was to establish both the level of dental health of Northern Ireland adults and their attitudes towards dental services, a representative sample of this group was required. For the purposes of the survey adults were defined as those aged 16 and over. People living in institutions, that is school boarders, residential students, people in hostels and hospitals, convalescent and old peoples' homes etc were excluded from the survey coverage because of the many practical difficulties of interviewing their residents and the difficult sampling problems they present.

2.2 The Electoral Register

To obtain a representative sample of the defined group it is necessary to have a complete list of all adults resident in Northern Ireland. Theoretically the Electoral Register is such a list and permission was granted by the Chief Electoral Officer to use this for the selection of the sample. Two problems arise with the use of the Electoral Register as a sampling frame, one on a general level, affecting all surveys and the other specifically related to the scope of this survey. On the general level it is known that for reasons such as people moving home and deaths between compilation dates, the register is not entirely up to date. To compensate for this a supplementary sampling procedure was used. On the specific level the Electoral Register lists people of 18 years and upwards yet this survey is based on 16 years of age and upwards. Again the supplementary sampling procedure was used to compensate.

2.3 The Supplementary Sampling Procedure

Interviewers were provided with address sheets on which all adults registered at the selected addresses were written. A number 1 was marked opposite the name of the person to be interviewed. On tracing the selected person, interviewers showed the list of names to the respondent and asked if there were any other adults, aged 16 or over, living at that address who were not on the list. If there were, the extra names were listed in the order given beneath those already on the sheet.

The next problem then was to ascertain which, if any, of these extra people to interview. To do this a line was drawn across the address sheet at the bottom of the list of names from the Electoral Register, and the extra people at the address listed immediately beneath that line. Of those names above the line, if the second name was selected for interview then the second name below the line was also selected for interview; if it was the first above the line, then it was the first below the line. Equally, if the fourth named person had been interviewed and there were only two extra inhabitants no extra interview would be carried out. In this way 16 and 17 year olds and any other adults not listed by the Electoral Register were selected for interview.

A similar exercise was undertaken when the listed family no longer lived at that address. The new occupants were listed below the line and the same selection procedure adopted. Outcome boxes were also provided beside the names so that interviewers could specify whether or not an interview was achieved, and if not, the reason for non-contact.

2.4 Selecting the Sample

To ensure that the selected sample adequately represented all areas in Northern Ireland a three stage sampling procedure was used, yielding a random sample of approximately 1,500 names.

Stage one: Health and Social Services Boards

The proportions of the total population living in each of the 4 Health and Social Services Board Areas were calculated to ensure that the same proportions were reflected in the survey sample. This was to ensure that valid comparisons could therefore be made in respect of dental health in each Board.

Stage two: the selection of wards

Within each Health Board Area the wards were listed in order of increasing household density ie households (number of domestic properties on the valuation list) per hectare. Wards were then selected by probability according to electoral size, being chosen by taking a random start and constant interval where:

$$\text{constant interval} = \frac{\text{total number of electors in Board Area}}{\text{number of wards to be selected.}}$$

Altogether 120 wards were chosen in this way.

Stage three: the selection of individuals

The number of persons per ward to be selected varied according to Health Board Area size. Again, a random start began the selection coupled with a constant interval.

Altogether 1,517 names and addresses were selected for interview. Due to the lower refusal rate amongst housewives in the selected sample, it was decided to examine these as a separate group for certain parts of the survey.

2.5   Obtaining the Information

Interviewers on completing an introductory questionnaire which ascertained the informant's dental state went on to complete the main questionnaire. Yellow (No. 1) questionnaires were for people with only natural teeth; green (No. 3) questionnaires for the edentulous; and pink (No. 2) questionnaires for those with a combination of natural teeth and dentures. At the end of the interview a supplementary questionnaire looking into the availability of dental services in Northern Ireland was completed. Those informants who had some natural teeth were then asked if they could be examined by a dentist and if they were agreeable an appointment was arranged for as soon as possible after the interview. Interviewers were instructed to make the dental appointment within one week of the interview day to reduce the chances of altered clinical condition between interview and examination and also to reduce the likelihood of broken examination appointments. Copies of the questionnaires and examination chart can be seen at Appendix 4 and Appendix 6.

It was regarded as impractical to combine the interview and the examination in one visit. The presence of the dentist could have influenced the informants replies to the questionnaire and could have seemed to imply expectation of consent to the dental examination which was intended to be voluntary. More seriously, combining interview and examination could have caused much of the dentists' time to be wasted.

2.6   Minimising Non-Contact

In order to minimise the possibility of non-contact, interviewers called to the selected addresses at several different times of the day. In general the contact rate was high despite difficulties caused by persons having moved away or premises being abandoned. Taking changed addresses into consideration 86% of persons listed were interviewed.

2.7   The Interview

The 3 interview schedules were the same as those used in the UK Adult Dental Health Survey of 1978 (Appendix 4). An additional schedule used in Northern Ireland only was added (Appendix 4).

One questionnaire was relevant to persons having no natural teeth (No. 3 schedule), one to those wearing partial dentures (No. 2 schedule) and one to those with natural teeth only (No. 1 schedule). The Northern Ireland schedule of questions was relevant to all persons seeking health service dental treatment. The total time taken to complete questionnaires varied between thirty-five and fifty minutes.

2.8   The Dental Examination

All the dental examinations were carried out at the informants place of residence. In order to ensure that lighting was standardised, each dental examiner was issued with portable mouth lights and probes similar to those used in the UK Adult Dental Health Survey of 1978. The informant sat in an ordinary household chair. The dentist stored the mirrors and instruments in an alcoholic solution of chlorhexidine.

In order to cause the least possible disturbance or inconvenience to the informants each dentist carried hand cleansing facilities.

It would have been undesirable for any of the dental examiners to have become involved in discussions about the informants dental health. For that reason, the dentists name was not used and the interviewer who was acting as the recorder attempted to prevent the dentist entering into any discussions with the informant.

6

2.9 Content of the Dental Examination

The criteria used in the survey were the same as those used in the UK Adult Dental Health Survey of 1978. The dental conditions which were recorded are listed in Appendix 6 and the criteria for recording the conditions are listed in Appendix 5.

2.10 Training of the Dental Examiners

Each dental examiner attended a calibration course to ensure standardisation of results and to reduce examiner variability as much as possible. A copy of the criteria for the examination (Appendix 5) was sent to each examiner prior to the calibration course to familiarise the examiner with the criteria.

A series of exercises recording clinical findings from models, slides and mounted teeth made up the first part of the course.

The dental examiners recorded their findings, comparison was made with defined standards and any discrepancies identified.

The examiners spent two days on exercises, examining and reporting on various dental conditions before commencing clinical training.

The examiners commenced the clinical part of the course by working in groups of three. One dentist acted as examiner, one as examinee and one as recorder. Dental findings were recorded on the charts to be used in the survey. All charts were collected, scrutinised by tutors and any discrepancies brought to the attention of the examiner. The third and part of the fourth day were spent in working in groups of three. The rest of the fourth day was spent in examining volunteers with one dentist as examiner and the other as recorder.

On the last day of the course, the dental examiners and the dental recorders met for the first time. Some time was spent recording conditions from charts which had been completed previously. This gave the recorders extra practice in recording and also permitted them to become accustomed to the sound of the voices of the dentists with whom they would be working. After further practice recording the oral condition of volunteers, the reproducibility examinations were recorded. The oral conditions of a selected group of volunteers were examined and recorded. The same group returned for examinations when the survey was complete. The results of the reproducibility examinations are shown in Appendix 7.

3. Public Response to the Survey

Surveys which depend upon a voluntary response from the public can provide inadequate information if the persons selected for the sample do not co-operate. An adult dental health survey requiring completion of a lengthy questionnaire followed by a dental examination requires a very high level of public co-operation.

Some persons though willing to co-operate in providing information for questionnaires may be reluctant to permit a dental examination. In order to overcome any such reluctance the interviewer was able to reassure such persons that the same interviewer would return at the time of examination and act as recorder. The interviewer could also explain that the examination was a simple rapid one causing no discomfort or inconvenience.

3.1 Non-response

Non-response in any survey is a cause for concern since one particular group may well be under represented. The refusal rate in particular can be a reflection of the acceptability of the survey to the public since it shows those people who are contacted and yet decline to take part in the survey. The fact that only 35 people or 2% of those eligible refused to be interviewed illustrates both the ease of interview and the level of interest in the subject of the public at large.

Besides those who refused to take part in the survey there are also those whom the interviewers were unable to contact because they were unavailable for interview for a variety of reasons (away all survey period, never in, too ill, handicapped etc). The case of no eligible person at a household arose where one family had moved out, another had moved in and on completing the sampling procedure, no-one's name fell on a numbered line. All in all unavoidable losses brought the non-contact rate up to a total of 14% leaving an initial response rate of 86%—a rate similar to previous Adult Dental Health studies in England and Wales (1968) and Scotland (1972).

Response rate for the dental examination at 76% was comparable to the above studies and very favourable for an examination of such a personal nature.

TABLE 3.1

Response to the Survey

Initial sample	1,517	
Dead	10	
Vacant/derelict	39	
Institutions	2	
No eligible person/no longer lives at address	91	
Eligible addresses	1,375	
		Response rate
Interviews carried out:		
People who have/had Partial Dentures (Schedule 2)	231 ⎫	
People with Natural Teeth Only (Schedule 1)	552 ⎬ Dentate	
People with No Natural Teeth (Schedule 3)	393 ⎭ Edentulous	
TOTAL	1,176	86%
Refusals	35	2%
General non contact	127	9%
Out all calls	24	2%
Away all survey	13	1%
Examination Response Rate:		
No. of people eligible	783	
No. examined	592	76%

3.2 Definition of Terms*

Throughout this report certain terms are used which should be explained at the outset to avoid confusion.

    (i) Social class. The social classification scheme used was the Registrar General's Classification of Occupations (1970).

    (ii) Health Board. Addresses were categorised into whichever of the 4 Northern Ireland Health and Social Services Boards they were situated in.

    (iii) Age. Informants were asked for their date of birth and had their ages calculated using 1 September 1979 (start date of fieldwork interviewing) as the base.

    (iv) Base numbers reweighted. At the bottom of many tables the terms "base numbers reweighted" appears. This means that the percentages shown in each of these tables is calculated using the numbers to whom that particular question applied as a base. This also explains why totals sometimes vary from one table to the next. For example a question asking whether or not a person cleans his/her teeth would have an answer from all the sample, whereas one asking what he/she cleans the teeth with would only apply to those who clean them.

---

*The definition of terms is included here, less because it relates to public response than because it immediately precedes the survey findings.

4. Persons with no Natural Teeth

One indicator of the dental health of a community is the number of adults with no natural teeth. The proportion of the adult population which was totally edentulous was identified in the UK Adult Dental Health Surveys of 1968 (England and Wales) and 1972 (Scotland). The percentages varied not only between countries but between age groups, social class and the sexes. Changing attitudes to dental health and the availability of dental services can be reflected in the proportion of the population who are edentulous. The England and Wales Survey of 1968 showed that more than 45% of the persons who had lost all their natural teeth had lost them before the Health Service began. The results of the UK Adult Dental Health Survey of 1978 and the Northern Ireland Adult Dental Health Survey of 1979 are shown in Table 4.1.

TABLE 4.1

Proportion of People with No Natural Teeth in England and Wales and in Northern Ireland.
The results of the United Kingdom* and Northern Ireland surveys compared.

Present Age	Male %		Female %		All %	
	E/W	NI	E/W	NI	E/W	NI
16–34	3	2	4	5	3	3.5
35–44	9	15	14	19	12	17
45–54	24	22	33	37	29	35
55–64	41	51	56	74	48	64
65–74	72	71	76	64	74	67
75 and over . . .	86	65	87	77	87	74
All Ages	24	30	32	37	29	33

4.1 Total Tooth Loss and Household Social Class

The proportion of persons with no natural teeth varied according to household social class. Household social class was determined by the occupation of the head of the household. The housewife category was largely comprised of the elderly which is the reason for the high percentage of edentulousness in this group. There was a wide variation in the degree of edentulousness between the non-manual classes (16%) and the manual semi-skilled and unskilled classes (47%), (Table 4.2).

TABLE 4.2

Total Tooth Loss by Household Social Class

Household Social Class	Proportion edentulous
I Professional	
II Managerial	16%
III Non-manual skilled	
III Manual skilled	18%
IV Non-manual semi-skilled . . .	19%
IV Manual semi-skilled	
V Unskilled	47%
Housewife	50%
Others	43

*Adult Dental Health Vol. 1: England and Wales 1968–1978. J. E. Todd, A. M. Walker. HMSO 1980.

5. Adults with Some Natural Teeth

In any survey of adult dental health one aspect of interest which emerges is the perception of the individual of his or her own dental health status and needs.

Persons who had some natural teeth of their own were asked the same series of questions whether or not they wore a partial denture. The replies permitted some assessment to be made of the dental health of the informant even before the dental examination.

The proportion of persons with some natural teeth who had suffered from toothache within the four weeks prior to the interview was 9%. During the same four weeks 10% had lost fillings or had lost pieces of tooth. 6% thought that they had some loose teeth and 15% avoided using certain teeth when eating or drinking. The most common reason for avoiding the teeth was because cavities in the teeth caused toothache.

The proportion who thought that they had some decayed teeth was 40%.

As disease of the gums is just as important in terms of dental health as disease of the teeth, the interview contained questions relating to the gums. 3% thought that their gums were swollen at the time of interview. Persons interviewed were asked whether they thought that they would require treatment if they were to visit the dentist the following day. 60% said that they thought that they would require treatment and 40% said that they would not.

The dental examination established the presence or absence of teeth. Teeth present were classified as follows:—

Missing	Filled but decayed
Unrestorable	Filled otherwise sound
Decayed (not previously treated)	Sound and untreated

The full complement of natural teeth is 32 and each tooth was listed in only one of the categories.

TABLE 5.1

Average Number of Sound, Decayed and Treated Teeth among Adults with Some Natural Teeth

Tooth Conditions	Average number of teeth in each condition								
	Adults aged 16–34 with some natural teeth			Adults aged 35 or over with some natural teeth			Adults of all ages with some natural teeth		
	Male	Female	Total	Male	Female	Total	Male	Female	Total
Sound and untreated	14.4	12.6	13.4	10.3	8.8	9.5	12.2	10.7	11.4
Crowned or bridged	0.4	0.4	0.4	0.2	0.3	0.3	0.3	0.4	0.3
Filled otherwise sound . . .	8.8	10.2	9.5	5.9	8.6	7.3	7.2	9.4	8.4
Filled and decayed	0.7	0.7	0.7	0.5	0.5	0.5	0.6	0.6	0.6
Decayed, untreated but restorable .	1.2	0.8	1.0	1.1	0.5	0.8	1.2	0.6	0.9
Unrestorable	0.3	0.3	0.3	0.5	0.1	0.3	0.4	0.2	0.3
Missing	6.2	7.2	6.8	13.4	13.1	13.2	10.1	10.1	10.1
Total	32.0	32.0	32.0	32.0	32.0	32.0	32.0	32.0	32.0
Base	128	163	291	146	155	301	274	318	592

NOTE: In this chapter, the category "teeth present" includes all crowns. The category "teeth at risk" does not.

5.1 Decayed, Missing and Filled Teeth

One simple way of estimating dental health from the results of a survey such as this is to measure the number of decayed, missing and filled teeth. A total number of these teeth gives a round figure for each individual. Thus the higher the figure, the worse the dental health.

Such figures are useful for making comparisons between one survey area and another. An average DMF(T) figure for one area can provide a basis for comparison with another provided that the examination conditions and criteria are similar. Such estimates are convenient but are at best crude assessments of dental health. More accurate evaluations require more precise measurements.

TABLE 5.2

The Number of Decayed Teeth for Adults with Some Natural Teeth

Number of teeth in each condition	Unrestorable teeth	Decayed teeth (not previously treated)	Filled but decayed teeth	Total decayed teeth
	%	%	%	%
0	86	64	65	43
1– 2	11	23	29	31
3– 5	2	10	5	19
6– 8	1	2	1	5
9–11	—	1	—	2
12 or more	*	—	—	*
Average number of teeth in each condition	0.3	0.9	0.6	1.7
BASE		592		

Base number re-weighted.
*Less than 0.5%.

These figures indicate a considerable amount of treatment need. Even though the dental examination did not measure early decay, half of the people with some natural teeth had between one and five decayed teeth requiring treatment.

On average, adults in Northern Ireland with some natural teeth had 19.8 teeth free from decay. Not all of these teeth, of course, had always been decay-free; 42% of the 19.8 had been decayed, the decay having been treated so that these teeth were sound at the time of the dental examination.

Perhaps even more interesting than the average number of teeth in these conditions is the variation in the number of teeth in these conditions. Nearly half (49%) of adults who still had some natural teeth had 9 or more that were filled, otherwise sound. (Table 5.3).

In terms of the number of teeth that were sound and untreated it is obvious that very few people in the community have the good fortune to maintain a full and healthy dentition without the intervention of the dentist. Although our sample included adults from the age of sixteen, only 6% of those with some natural teeth had 21 or more teeth that were sound and untreated.

TABLE 5.3

The Number of Sound Teeth for Adults with Some Natural Teeth

Number of teeth in each condition	Adults with some natural teeth	
	Filled, otherwise sound teeth	Sound and untreated teeth
	%	%
0	13	1
1– 2	8	3
3– 5	12	10
6– 8	18	20
9–11	17	19
12–14	15	20
15–17	11	14
18–20	5	7
21–23	1	5
24–26	—	1
27 or more	—	*
Average number of teeth in each condition	8.4	11.4
BASE	592	592

*Less than 0.5%.

The tooth conditions have been shown separately. For interest the various conditions are shown together, in order to compare their relative importance. Table 5.4 therefore gives in summary, for adults of all ages with some natural teeth, the distribution of the major tooth conditions.

TABLE 5.4

The Number of Teeth in the Different Conditions for Adults with Some Natural Teeth

Number of teeth in each condition	Adults with some natural teeth			
	Missing teeth	Decayed teeth	Filled, otherwise sound teeth	Sound and untreated teeth
	%	%	%	%
0	2	43	13	1
1– 5	26	50	20	13
6–11	40	7	35	39
12–17	16	0	25	33
18 or more	16	0	7	14
	100	100	100	100
Average number of teeth in each condition	10.1	1.7	8.4	11.4
BASE	592	592	592	592

Base number re-weighted.

On average, adults of all ages who still had some natural teeth had 10.1 that were missing, 1.7 that were decayed, 8.4 filled, otherwise sound, and 11.4 that were sound and untreated.

5.2 The Condition of the Natural Teeth by Age

Total tooth loss varies with age, sex and social class. These factors also relate to dental health among those people who still have some of their natural teeth. The condition of the natural teeth in relation to age, sex and social class are thus shown in Table 5.5. The numbers of dentate adults in the oldest age groups are fairly small. All people aged 55 and over are grouped together.

Tooth loss varies with age, and this is shown by Table 5.5, the average number of missing teeth increasing steadily with age from 5.1 among those aged 16–24 to 17.3 among those aged 55 and over. In this oldest age group half of the people who still had some natural teeth had lost 18 or more, ie more than half of their natural teeth. Only a very small proportion of people had a full complement of 32 teeth; Table 5.5 shows that a consistent small proportion of each age group had 32 natural teeth present, with the youngest age group more likely to have all their teeth.

TABLE 5.5

The Number of Missing Teeth for Adults of Different Ages

Number of missing teeth	Adults with some natural teeth					
	16–24	25–34	35–44	45–54	55 and over	All ages
	%	%	%	%	%	%
0	4	2	1	0	1	2
1– 5	54	26	20	15	3	26
6–11	40	49	44	37	22	40
12–17	2	18	15	33	24	16
18 or more	0	5	20	15	50	16
	100	100	100	100	100	100
Average number of missing teeth	5.1	8.5	11.1	11.7	17.3	10.1
BASES	144	143	123	86	96	592

Base numbers re-weighted.

In Tables 5.6 and 5.7 we give the figures separately for those who rely wholly on natural teeth and those who have a denture, these two groups having been found to differ markedly in the numbers of missing teeth.

13

Carrying out analyses by the combination of age and dental status results in the numbers in some of the groups being rather small; particularly small are the number of partially-dentured people in the age group 16–24. Despite the small numbers, the steady increase of tooth loss with age as shown by the average number of missing teeth can still be seen. Of course, age for age, those people with dentures had considerably more missing teeth than those with no dentures. For example, if we consider the proportions of people having 18 or more missing teeth, this was a rare occurrence among adults who rely wholly on natural teeth (even in our oldest age group only 20% had this number of teeth missing), whereas among those who have natural teeth and dentures considerable numbers had this level of tooth loss.

TABLE 5.6

The Number of Missing Teeth for Adults of Different Ages who Rely Wholly on Natural Teeth

Number of missing teeth	Adults who rely wholly on natural teeth					
	Present age					All ages
	16–24	25–34	35–44	45–44	55 and over	
	%	%	%	%	%	%
0	4	3	1	—	3	3
1– 5	55	31	31	24	5	35
6–11	40	50	55	44	42	46
12–17	1	16	11	30	30	13
18 or more	—	—	2	2	20	3
	100	100	100	100	100	100
Average number of missing teeth .	5.0	7.2	7.9	9.1	13.0	7.4
BASES	139	117	75	54	40	425

TABLE 5.7

The Number of Missing Teeth for Adults of Different Ages with Some Natural Teeth who have a Denture

Number of missing teeth	Adults with some natural teeth who have a denture					
	Present age					All ages
	16–24	25–34	35–44	45–54	55 and over	
	%	%	%	%	%	%
0	—	—	—	—	—	—
1– 5	40	4	4	—	2	4
6–11	60	42	27	25	7	23
12–17	—	27	21	37	20	24
18 or more	—	27	48	38	71	49
	100	100	100	100	100	100
Average number of missing teeth .	6.6	14.2	16.1	16.1	20.4	17.0
BASES	5	26	48	32	56	167

Base numbers re-weighted.

This large variation of tooth loss with age must be borne in mind in the following analyses of the different conditions of the teeth present; the older people had considerably fewer teeth present (and therefore "at risk") than younger people, ie fewer teeth which could be decayed, filled, or sound.

Next to be considered are those teeth which were found to be decayed, and Table 5.8 gives the distribution of decayed teeth for adults of different ages.

14

TABLE 5.8

The Number of Decayed Teeth for Adults of Different Ages

Number of decayed teeth	Adults with some natural teeth					
	Present age					All ages
	16–24	25–34	35–44	45–54	55 and over	
	%	%	%	%	%	%
0	44	37	43	43	51	43
1– 5	46	55	54	55	39	50
6–11	9	8	3	2	9	7
12 or more	1	0	0	0	1	0
	100	100	100	100	100	100
Average number of decayed teeth .	2.0	1.8	1.4	1.4	1.9	1.7
Average number of teeth present .	26.9	23.5	20.9	20.3	14.7	21.9
BASES	144	143	123	86	96	592

Base numbers re-weighted.

Decayed teeth were not confined to any particular age group or groups. There was some variation in the decay average between age groups. For example 10% of those aged 16–24 had 6 or more currently decayed teeth compared to only 2% of those aged 45–54.

As discussed earlier the measurement of decay was defined from three categories of decay, that is teeth which are unrestorable, those that are decayed (not previously treated) and those which have been filled but are now also decayed. It is of interest to examine the average number of teeth that are decayed in each age group to see whether the contributions being made by the different kinds of decay are constant for all ages. Table 5.9 shows the average broken down into its component parts.

People in the oldest age group had, on average, slightly more unrestorable teeth, although teeth in this condition did occur even among the youngest people. The number of filled teeth which were now decayed was fairly constant for all age groups, but teeth which were decayed, and not yet unrestorable, but which had no signs of previous treatment were somewhat more prevalent among both the youngest and the oldest adults.

TABLE 5.9

The Average Number of Decayed Teeth for Adults of Different Ages

Average number of teeth which were:	Adults with some natural teeth					
	Present age					All ages
	16–24	25–34	35–44	45–54	55 and over	
Unrestorable	0.3	0.2	0.2	0.1	0.5	0.3
Decayed, not previously treated .	1.1	0.8	0.6	0.7	1.1	0.8
Filled but decayed	0.6	0.8	0.6	0.3	0.3	0.6
Total decayed teeth . . .	2.0	1.8	1.4	1.4	1.9	1.7
Average number of teeth present .	26.9	23.5	20.9	20.3	14.7	21.9
BASES	144	143	123	86	96	592

Table 5.10 gives the distribution of the number of teeth which had at one time been decayed but had been filled so that they were sound at the time of the dental examination.

15

Table 5.10

The Number of Filled, Otherwise Sound Teeth for Adults of Different Ages

Number of filled, otherwise sound teeth	Adults with some natural teeth					
	Present age					All ages
	16–24	25–34	35–44	45–54	55 and over	
	%	%	%	%	%	%
0	6	7	11	15	35	13
1– 5	17	16	18	17	33	20
6–11	38	41	36	36	20	35
12–17	32	30	21	28	10	25
18 or more	7	6	14	4	2	7
	100	100	100	100	100	100
Average number of filled, otherwise sound teeth	9.5	9.5	9.1	8.3	4.2	8.4
Average number of teeth present	26.9	23.5	20.9	20.3	14.7	21.9
BASES	144	143	123	86	96	592

The people in the oldest age group, those aged 55 and over, had on average 4.9* fewer teeth that were filled, otherwise sound, than other people, but of course these older people had fewer teeth at risk. The variation in the number of filled, otherwise sound teeth occurred in the older age groups. Among the youngest adults 6% had no teeth which were filled, otherwise sound and 39% had 12 or more filled teeth. In the oldest age group, 35% had no teeth which were filled and only 12% had 12 or more filled teeth.

In Table 5.1 it was shown that adults had, on average, 11.4 teeth which had remained free from decay. Table 5.11 shows that as a general trend the average number of teeth in this condition declines with age, from 15.0 teeth among those aged 16–24, to 8.1 teeth among those aged 55 and over.

Table 5.11

The Number of Sound and Untreated Teeth for Adults of Different Ages

Number of sound and untreated teeth	Adults with some natural teeth					
	Present age					All ages
	16–24	25–34	35–44	45–54	55 and over	
	%	%	%	%	%	%
0	—	1	1	2	2	1
1– 5	1	8	17	12	30	13
6–11	22	39	49	45	48	39
12–17	49	37	26	33	16	33
18 or more	28	15	7	8	4	14
	100	100	100	100	100	100
Average number of sound and untreated teeth	15.0	11.8	9.9	10.5	8.1	11.4
Average number of teeth present	26.9	23.5	20.9	20.3	14.7	21.9
BASES	144	143	123	86	96	592

As we would expect, only a small proportion of people in this oldest age group had a large number of sound and untreated teeth (4% had 18 or more); but even in our youngest age group, less than one third of the people had 18 or more teeth which had always been decay-free.

In Table 5.12 we summarise and give the average number of teeth in each of the main conditions for adults of different ages.

---

*Average of the differences between the oldest and the other age groups.

It must be remembered that, as mentioned above, the number of teeth in different conditions is influenced by the levels of tooth loss. This is particularly pertinent in the older age groups where there are high levels of tooth loss. For instance, those people aged 55 and over would appear to be better off in terms of decayed teeth than those aged 16–24 (these two groups having on average 1.9 and 2.0 decayed teeth respectively). But the people in the oldest age group had only 14.2 teeth "at risk", compared to 26.5 among those aged 16–24.

TABLE 5.12

The Average Number of Teeth in the Different Conditions for Adults of Different Ages

Average number of teeth which were:	Adults with some natural teeth					
	Present age					All ages
	16–24	25–34	35–44	45–54	55 and over	
Missing	5.1	8.5	11.1	11.7	17.3	10.1
Present	26.9	23.5	20.9	20.3	14.7	21.9
	32.0	32.0	32.0	32.0	32.0	32.0
Decayed	2.0	1.8	1.4	1.4	1.9	1.7
Filled (otherwise sound) . .	9.5	9.5	9.1	8.3	4.2	8.4
Sound and untreated . . .	15.0	11.8	9.9	10.5	8.1	11.4
(Teeth at risk)	26.5	23.1	20.4	20.2	14.2	21.5
BASES	144	143	123	86	96	592

In Table 5.13 the distributions and averages for the main tooth conditions are shown separately for men and for women.

5.3 The Condition of the Natural Teeth by Sex

TABLE 5.13

The Number of Teeth in the Different Conditions for Men and Women

Number of teeth in each condition	Adults with some natural teeth							
	Missing teeth		Decayed teeth		Filled teeth		Sound and untreated teeth	
	M	F	M	F	M	F	M	F
	%	%	%	%	%	%	%	%
0	3	1	38	48	19	8	1	2
1– 5	24	28	51	49	34	32	10	15
6–11	39	41	11	3	23	21	37	41
12–17	20	13	*	—	20	29	36	31
18 or more	14	17	—	*	4	10	16	11
	100	100	100	100	100	100	100	100
Average number of teeth in each condition	10.1	10.1	2.2	1.4	7.2	9.4	12.2	10.7
BASES	274	318	274	318	274	318	274	318

*Less than 0.4%.

There was greater evidence of dental treatment, and particularly restorative treatment, among women than among men, women having on average 2.2 more that were filled, otherwise sound, than men. Only 8% of women had no filled teeth compared to 19% of men. Large numbers of filled teeth were more often found among women, 39% having 12 or more filled, otherwise sound teeth compared with 24% of men with that number of filled teeth.

Men on the other hand more frequently had teeth with active decay, only 38% of men having no decayed teeth compared with 48% of women. On average the men had nearly 1 more decayed tooth. The men were also more likely to have a greater number of teeth classified as sound and untreated; on average they had more teeth in this condition than did the women. In fact 89% of men had 6 or more sound and untreated teeth, whereas this was only so for 83% of the women.

17

The pattern of dentures in combination with natural teeth varies somewhat for men and women and this obviously is very closely related to which natural teeth were still at risk at the time of the dental examination and consequently to the numbers of teeth in the different conditions (see Chapter 7).

In Table 5.14 the tooth conditions for men and women of different ages are shown. When the tooth conditions are examined by more than one factor at once, a table giving the full distributions becomes unmanageable. On the other hand the averages alone give insufficient information. In some of the subsequent tables, instead of giving the full distribution, the proportions of people with certain numbers of teeth in the various conditions are shown.

Table 5.14 shows that the sex differences which were shown in Table 5.13 are in general true whatever age group is considered. It is of particular interest to examine the two youngest age groups, that is those aged 16–24 and those aged 25–34. Among the youngest adults (16–24), there was little (0.7) difference in the overall average number of missing teeth. There was however a difference in the amount of restorative treatment among the youngest adults, women having on average 2.2 more filled, otherwise sound teeth. The proportion of women in this age group who had no filled, otherwise sound teeth was lower (3% compared to 10% among the men), and the proportion of women who had 12 or more filled, otherwise sound teeth was higher (46% compared to only 31% among the men). In terms of decay among the youngest adults, there was a difference (1.2 teeth) between the sexes in the average number of teeth which were currently decayed, but proportionately more women were decay-free (54% compared to 34% among the men). The youngest men had on average almost 1.9 more sound and untreated teeth than the women.

In the next age group (25–34), there were again differences in the amount of restorative treatment, women having more filled, otherwise sound teeth than men. In addition there was in this age group some tooth loss difference between men and women, both in the average number of missing teeth and in the proportion who had 18 or more missing teeth. The women had on average 0.8 more missing teeth than the men, and 6% of the women had lost 18 or more natural teeth compared to only 3% among the men. Men had on average 1.4 more teeth that were sound and untreated. Decay levels however were almost exactly the same.

There is, therefore, evidence of more dental treatment having been undergone by the women, and more treatment need among the men, even among the youngest groups of adults.

TABLE 5.14

The Number of Teeth in the Different Conditions for Men and Women of Different Ages

Average number of teeth which were:	Adults with some natural teeth											
	16–24		25–34		35–44		45–54		55 and over		All ages	
	M	F	M	F	M	F	M	F	M	F	M	F
Missing . . .	4.7	5.4	8.0	8.8	10.2	11.9	12.2	11.1	18.6	16.2	10.1	10.1
Present . . .	27.3	26.6	24.0	23.2	21.8	20.1	19.8	20.9	13.4	15.8	21.9	21.9
Decayed . . .	2.6	1.4	1.8	1.9	1.8	1.1	1.8	1.1	2.8	1.0	2.2	1.4
Filled* . . .	8.4	10.6	9.2	9.8	7.6	10.3	7.2	9.5	2.4	5.8	7.2	9.4
Sound and untreated .	16.0	14.1	12.6	11.2	12.0	8.2	10.6	10.3	7.8	8.4	12.2	10.7
(Teeth at risk) . .	27.0	26.1	23.6	22.9	21.4	19.6	19.6	20.9	13.0	15.2	21.6	21.5
	%		%		%		%		%		%	
Proportion of people with:												
18 or more missing teeth	0	0	3	6	14	25	13	18	53	47	15	17
No decayed teeth . .	34	54	39	36	46	40	37	50	33	67	38	48
No filled* teeth . .	10	3	9	6	14	8	17	13	56	18	19	8
12 or more filled* teeth	31	46	31	41	23	45	22	42	7	16	24	39
BASES . . .	68	76	59	84	56	67	46	40	45	51	274	318

*Filled, otherwise sound.

5.4 The Condition of the Natural Teeth by Social Class

Table 5.15 gives the average number of teeth in the different conditions and certain indicators of dental health for different social classes.

11% of those in the top social class group had lost 18 or more teeth compared to 20% in the intermediate social class group and 17% in the lowest social class group. There were, however, considerable social class differences in the conditions of those teeth which were present, and it was the top social class group (ie professional, managerial and skilled non-manual grouped together) which was outstanding. These people had considerably more evidence of restorative treatment than people in the other two social class groups. For example they had higher numbers of filled teeth, only 8% of them had no filled teeth compared to 18% and 13% in the other two social class groups, and over one third of them (42%) had 12 or more filled teeth compared to 21% and 17% in the other two social class groups.

18

TABLE 5.15

The Number of Teeth in the Different Conditions for Different Social Classes

Average number of teeth which were:	Adults with some natural teeth				
	Household Social Class				All† Social Classes
	I, II and III non-manual	III manual	IV and V	Housewife	
Missing	8.7	11.4	10.8	11.2	10.1
Present	23.3	20.6	21.2	20.8	21.9
	32.0	32.0	32.0	32.0	32.0
Decayed	1.4	1.9	2.0	1.7	1.7
Filled*	10.1	7.1	6.9	8.8	8.4
Sound and untreated	11.5	11.3	11.9	9.7	11.3
Teeth at risk	23.0	20.3	20.8	20.2	21.5
	%	%	%	%	%
Proportion of people with:					
18 or more missing teeth . . .	11	20	17	20	16
No decayed teeth	52	35	39	39	43
No filled* teeth	8	18	13	15	13
12 or more filled teeth . . .	62	21	17	38	32
BASES	193	130	89	117	592

*Filled, otherwise sound.
†Includes the student, unemployed and unclassifiable categories which are not included elsewhere in the table.

There was, however, a reversal of this social class difference when the number of sound and untreated teeth was considered. Adults in the lowest social class group had on average 0.4 more sound and untreated teeth than adults in the top social class group. This (at first sight unexpected) result must, however be interpreted with extreme caution. On its own, "the number of sound and untreated teeth" can be a somewhat misleading indicator because of the differences in methods used in survey data collection and the methods available for use in clinical treatment. The home examination detected visible decay only. In a clinical situation the dentist may detect hidden decay by X-ray, or may decide to treat an earlier stage of visible decay than we were counting as such. Because of this those groups of the community more exposed to dental treatment can appear to have fewer sound and untreated teeth according to our examination criteria. For this reason the lower social classes appear to be in an overall 'healthier' dental position with regard to sound and untreated teeth as an indicator of dental health must therefore be borne in mind whenever the number of teeth in this condition for different groups of people are under consideration.

Tooth conditions for adults of different social classes and ages are shown below. In previous tables with figures for different ages, five age groups have been examined. Because of the small numbers of people which would result if each of these five groups was subdivided into the three main social class groups, it has been necessary to use broader age groups, 16–34, 35–54 and 55 and over. The figures for these three age groups are given in Tables 5.16, 5.17 and 5.18 respectively.

People aged 16–34 are considered in Table 5.16. There were some differences in the number of missing teeth and there was considerably more evidence of restorative treatment among people of the top social class group. Those people had on average 10.8 filled teeth compared to 8.8 in the intermediate social class group and 7.5 in the lowest social class group. Only 3% of people in the top social class group had no filled teeth compared to 4% and 12% in the other two groups.

There was much less current decay among the young top social class group, 48% of these people having no decayed teeth compared to 35% in the intermediate group and 31% in the lowest social class group.

TABLE 5.16

The Number of Teeth in the Different Conditions for Adults Aged 16–34 of Different Social Classes

| Average number of teeth which were: | Adults aged 16–34 with some natural teeth | | | | |
| | Household Social Class | | | | All† Social Classes |
	I, II and III non-manual	III manual	IV and V	Housewife	
Missing	5.6	8.0	7.1	8.0	6.7
Present	26.4	24.0	24.9	24.0	25.3
	32.0	32.0	32.0	32.0	32.0
Decayed	1.5	1.9	2.5	2.2	1.9
Filled*	10.8	8.8	7.5	10.1	9.7
Sound and untreated	13.7	12.8	14.7	11.2	13.3
Teeth at risk	26.0	23.5	24.7	23.5	24.9
	%	%	%	%	%
Proportion of people with:					
18 or more missing teeth	0	5	2	3	2
No decayed teeth	48	35	31	32	40
No filled* teeth	3	4	12	10	6
12 or more filled* teeth	45	28	19	46	38
BASES	91	57	42	59	277

*Filled, otherwise sound.
†Includes the student, unemployed and unclassifiable categories which are not included elsewhere in the table.

Among the youngest adults (16–34) the variation with social class was already established.

TABLE 5.17

The Number of Teeth in the Different Conditions for Adults Aged 35–54 of Different Social Classes

| Average number of teeth which were: | Adults aged 35–54 with some natural teeth | | | | |
| | Household Social Class | | | | All† Social Classes |
	I, II and III non-manual	III manual	IV and V	Housewife	
Missing	9.6	11.7	13.2	12.2	11.3
Present	22.4	20.3	18.8	19.8	20.7
	32.0	32.0	32.0	32.0	32.0
Decayed	0.9	1.8	2.1	1.2	1.4
Filled*	11.0	7.3	6.6	9.5	8.8
Sound and untreated	10.0	11.0	9.8	8.9	10.1
Teeth at risk	21.9	20.1	18.5	19.6	20.3
	%	%	%	%	%
Proportion of people with:					
18 or more missing teeth	11	17	26	27	18
No decayed teeth	56	36	37	39	44
No filled* teeth	8	15	11	15	13
12 or more filled* teeth	51	19	17	39	33
BASES	75	52	35	33	203

*Filled, otherwise sound.
†Includes the student, unemployed and unclassifiable categories which are not included elsewhere in the table.

In the next age group, adults aged 35–54 (Table 5.17) the social class differences were even more marked, resulting in people in the top social class group having a higher standard of dental health—they had on average almost twice the number of filled, otherwise sound teeth (11.0 filled teeth compared to only 6.6 in the lowest social class group). They had 1.2 fewer currently decayed teeth and 56% were decay-free, compared to only 37% of people of the same age in the lowest social class group.

Among the oldest adults, that is those aged 55 and over (Table 5.18) the social class differences observed for the other two age groups are less clear cut. Age seems to over-rule class differences.

TABLE 5.18

The Number of Teeth in the Different Conditions for Adults Aged 55 and Over of Different Social Classes

Average number of teeth which were:	Adults aged 55 and over with some natural teeth				
	Household Social Class				All† Social Classes
	I, II and III non-manual	III manual	IV and V	Housewife	
Missing	16.3	20.0	17.0	17.5	17.6
Present	15.7	12.0	15.0	14.5	14.4
	32.0	32.0	32.0	32.0	32.0
Decayed	2.3	2.1	0.5	1.4	1.9
Filled*	4.9	1.9	5.3	5.1	4.1
Sound and untreated	8.3	7.9	8.6	7.2	8.0
Teeth at risk	15.5	11.9	14.4	13.7	14.0
	%	%	%	%	%
Proportion of people with:					
18 or more missing teeth . .	48	67	42	48	51
No decayed teeth . . .	52	33	75	56	50
No filled* teeth	26	67	25	24	36
12 or more filled* teeth . . .	11	5	8	16	11
BASES	27	21	12	25	94

Base numbers re-weighted.

*Filled, otherwise sound.

†Includes the student, unemployed and unclassifiable categories which are not included elsewhere in the table.

5.5 The Condition of the Natural Teeth by Dental Attendance Pattern

Dental treatment involves an interaction of patient and dentist; the amount of treatment which a person has is obviously affected by the dental attendance pattern. Treatment cannot be carried out if the person does not go to the dentist. Table 5.19 shows the proportion of people visiting the dentist for a regular check-up, an occasional check-up, or when they were having trouble.

TABLE 5.19

Dental Attendance Pattern for Adults with Some Natural Teeth

Attendance pattern	All adults with some natural teeth
	%
Regular check-up	40
Occasional check-up	12
Only when having trouble . . .	48
	100
BASE	592

Base number re-weighted.

Only 4 in 10 (40%) of adults with some natural teeth visited the dentist for a regular check-up; a further 12% went for an occasional check-up, and just under half (48%) only went when they were having trouble. These were the informants' opinions of their dental attendance patterns. Some idea of the frequency of visits associated with these answers can be formed, as during the interview, questions were asked about the length of time since the last visit to the dentist. The relationship between the two is examined.

TABLE 5.20

Length of Time Since Last Visit, by Dental Attendance Pattern, for Adults with Some Natural Teeth

Length of time since last went to the dentist	Adults with some natural teeth			
	Regular check-up	Occasional check-up	Only when having trouble	All
	%	% ·	%	%
Under treatment now	9	9	6	7
Less than 6 months	68	32	16	39
6 months, up to 1 year	17	40	15	19
More than 1, up to 2 years	4	14	14	10
More than 2, up to 3 years	2	3	18	10
More than 3, up to 5 years	0	1	15	7
More than 5, up to 10 years	0	1	13	6
More than 10 years	0	0	3*	2
	100	100	100	100
BASES	234	73	285	592

Base numbers re-weighted.
*Includes two persons who had never been to a dentist.

Of those people who said that they went to the dentist for a regular check-up 94% said they had been to the dentist in the year prior to the interview (the other 6% had last been to the dentist 1–3 years before the interview). Among those who only went when they were having trouble, 37% had been to the dentist in the year prior to the interview, a further 18% not having been for at least 3 years. There was a small proportion (3%) of irregular attenders (ie those who only went to the dentist when they were having trouble with their teeth) whose visits to the dentist were obviously very infrequent indeed, their last visit being more than 10 years before the interview. Those people who said that they went for an occasional check-up had, in general, last been to the dentist somewhat longer ago than the regular attenders, but not as long as those who only went when having trouble. There was, therefore, good agreement between the person's statement about the regularity of their dental attendance and their estimate of the length of time since they last went to the dentist, so we may with confidence use the opinion statements in looking at variations in attendance.

The dental condition varied considerably with age, sex and social class. The way in which patterns of dental attendance are related to dental condition was next investigated. For reasons of clarity the detailed distributions of the numbers of teeth in the various conditions are not shown as the tables would become unmanageable. Instead, the averages and various dental indicators are shown. Since denture wearers have been shown to have fewer natural teeth at risk, some of the information about dentures is anticipated by including the proportion of dentate adults who have a denture and also the proportion with a full upper denture.

TABLE 5.21

The Number of Teeth in the Different Conditions, by Dental Attendance Pattern

Average number of teeth which were:	Adults with some natural teeth			
	Regular check-up	Occasional check-up	Only when having trouble	All
Missing	8.5	8.3	11.9	10.1
Present	23.5	23.7	20.1	21.9
Decayed	0.8	1.8	2.5	1.7
Filled†	11.5	9.9	5.5	8.4
Sound and untreated	10.6	11.8	11.9	11.4
Teeth at risk	22.9	23.5	19.9	21.5
	%	%	%	%
Proportion of people with:				
18 or more missing teeth	11	10	22	16
No decayed teeth	59	37	32	43
No filled teeth†	1	6	26	13
12 or more filled teeth	50	38	16	32
Natural teeth and dentures . . .	27	16	33	28
Full upper denture	5	7	10	8
BASES	234	73	285	592

Base numbers re-weighted.
†Filled, otherwise sound.

Table 5.21 shows that the number of teeth in each condition was quite different for the different attendance patterns. Persons who went for a regular check-up had on average slightly more missing teeth than those who only went when they were having trouble (8.5 missing compared to 8.3). Large numbers of missing teeth, however, were comparatively rare among the regular attenders (only 11% had 18 or more teeth missing) whereas this was more common among the irregular attenders (22% had 18 or more teeth missing).

Decayed teeth were far less common among those who went for a regular check-up, these people having on average 0.8 decayed teeth compared to 2.5 among those who only went when they were having trouble. Among the irregular dental attenders, who made up almost half of all the people examined, there was therefore a considerable amount of treatment need; in fact only 32% of this group of people had decay-free mouths compared to over half (59%) of the regular attenders.

There were large differences in the amounts of restorative work, the regular dental attenders having on average 11.5 filled, otherwise sound, teeth compared to only 5.5 among those who only went when having trouble. Very few of the regular attenders had not experienced restorative treatment (only 1% had no teeth which were filled, otherwise sound) whereas among the irregular attenders a considerable proportion (26%) had no filled teeth.

Table 5.22 looks at different dental conditions for different ages and attendance patterns. In the youngest age group, the main differences were in the number of teeth decayed and filled.

TABLE 5.22

The Number of Teeth in the Different Conditions for Different Ages and Attendance Patterns

Average number of teeth which were:	Adults with some natural teeth							
	Present age						All ages	
	16–34		35–54		55 and over			
	Regular	Irregular	Regular	Irregular	Regular	Irregular	Regular	Irregular
Missing	6.1	7.2	9.4	13.0	14.4	18.7	8.5	11.1
Present (at risk) . . .	25.9	24.8	22.6	19.0	17.6	13.3	23.5	20.9
Decayed	0.8	2.6	0.9	1.9	0.4	2.6	0.8	2.4
Filled†	11.9	8.1	12.1	6.0	8.6	2.1	11.5	6.4
Sound and untreated . .	12.6	13.9	9.2	10.9	7.9	8.3	10.6	11.9
Teeth at risk . . .	25.3	24.6	22.2	18.8	16.9	13.0	22.9	20.7
	%	%	%	%	%	%	%	%
Proportion of people with:								
18 or more missing teeth . .	2	3	12	24	39	55	11	19
No decayed teeth . .	58	30	55	33	77	39	59	33
No filled teeth† . .	0	11	1	22	3	51	1	22
12 or more filled teeth . .	53	28	53	18	32	2	50	20
Natural teeth and dentures . .	11	11	32	44	65	55	27	29
Full upper denture . .	0	2	6	14	13	23	5	9
BASES	108	179	95	114	31	65	234	358

Base numbers re-weighted.

†Filled, otherwise sound.

Among those aged 35–54 there were again differences in decay, the regular attenders having on average 0.9 decayed teeth compared to 1.9 among the irregular attenders. Decay-free mouths were again much more common among the regular attenders than among the irregular attenders (the proportions with no decayed teeth were 55% and 33% respectively). The amount of restorative treatment differed markedly, the regular attenders having 12.1 teeth which were filled, otherwise sound, compared to only 6.0 among the irregular attenders (the proportions who had no filled, otherwise sound, teeth were 1% and 22% respectively, and the proportions with 12 or more were 53% and 18% respectively).

Among the oldest people, that is those aged 55 and over, the numbers of regular and irregular attenders were both small. Despite this, the difference within attendance pattern still existed, the regular attenders having on average fewer missing, fewer decayed, and more filled, otherwise sound teeth than the irregular attenders (in this age group the regular attenders had virtually the same number of sound and untreated teeth as the irregular attenders, but the regular attenders had far more teeth at risk than the irregular attenders).

Having seen earlier that there was some difference between men and women in dental condition, it is of interest to see whether or not regular dental attendance benefits the sexes alike; in Table 5.23 the position for males and females is shown separately. Because the numbers of people in the oldest age group, that is those aged 55 and over, were small, Table 5.23 shows only the age groups 16–34 and 35–54.

Among those aged 16–34 both among the regular and among the irregular attenders there were some sex differences. The men who were irregular attenders had on average 1.3 fewer missing teeth than the women; comparatively few of the men had high levels of tooth loss (2% had 18 or more teeth missing). The proportion among the female irregular attenders was 3%. Among these irregular attenders, the men had 1.6 more sound and untreated teeth and 0.8 fewer filled, otherwise sound, teeth.

In the next age group, 35–54, regular dental attendance benefitted the sexes similarly in that the male regular attenders had almost the same numbers of teeth in the different conditions as the female regular attenders. It is interesting that among those who only went to the dentist when having trouble, the difference in tooth loss between the sexes (which we observed for the youngest adults) was more marked among those aged 35–54. Although very few of the irregular attenders had extensive evidence of restorative treatment, among the female irregular attenders in this age group 20% had 12 or more filled teeth compared to only 16% of the male irregular attenders.

TABLE 5.23

The Number of Teeth in the Different Conditions for Different Sexes and Attendance Patterns

Average number of teeth which were:	Adults aged 16–34 with some natural teeth						Adults aged 35–54 with some natural teeth					
	Males		Females		Both		Males		Females		Both	
	Regular	Irregular	Regular	Irregular	Regular	Irregular	Regular	Irregular	Regular	Irregular	Regular	Irregular
Missing	5.7	6.5	6.4	7.8	6.1	7.2	9.4	11.9	9.4	14.7	9.4	13.0
Present (at risk)	26.3	25.5	25.6	24.2	25.9	24.8	22.6	20.1	22.6	17.3	22.6	19.0
Decayed	1.0	2.8	0.7	2.3	0.8	2.6	1.2	2.0	0.7	1.6	0.9	1.9
Filled*	10.9	7.7	12.5	8.5	11.9	8.1	11.2	5.7	12.5	6.4	12.1	6.0
Sound and untreated	13.8	14.7	11.9	13.1	12.6	13.9	9.7	12.1	8.9	9.0	9.2	10.9
Proportion of people with:	%	%	%	%	%	%	%	%	%	%	%	%
18 or more missing teeth	0	2	3	3	2	3	6	17	14	34	14	24
No decayed teeth	56	27	60	33	58	30	59	34	52	32	55	33
No filled* teeth	0	14	0	8	0	11	3	21	0	23	1	22
12 or more filled* teeth	44	24	58	32	53	28	38	16	60	20	53	18
Natural teeth and dentures	7	11	13	11	11	11	31	46	32	41	32	44
Full upper denture	0	1	0	2	0	2	3	6	8	28	6	14
BASES	41	86	67	93	108	179	32	70	63	44	95	114

Base numbers re-weighted.

*Filled, otherwise sound.

TABLE 5.24

The Number of Teeth in the Different Conditions for Different Social Classes, Sexes and Attendance Patterns

Average number of teeth which were	Adults aged 16–34 with some natural teeth									
	Household Social Class								All Social* Classes	
	I, II and III non-manual		III manual		IV non-manual, IV Manual and V		Housewife			
	Regular	Irregular	Regular	Irregular	Regular	Irregular	Regular	Irregular	Regular	Irregular
Missing	5.2	6.1	7.5	8.2	8.0	6.7	6.6	8.6	6.1	7.1
Present	26.8	25.9	24.5	23.8	24.0	25.3	25.4	23.4	25.9	24.9
Decayed	0.6	2.3	1.4	2.1	1.2	2.9	0.8	2.9	0.8	2.6
Filled†	12.3	9.5	9.9	8.4	11.2	6.3	14.3	8.1	11.9	8.3
Sound and untreated	13.6	13.9	12.6	12.9	10.9	16.0	9.2	12.2	12.6	13.8
Teeth at risk	26.5	25.7	23.9	23.4	23.3	25.2	24.3	23.2	25.3	24.7
Proportion of people with:	%	%	%	%	%	%	%	%	%	%
18 or more missing teeth	0	0	6	5	9	0	0	5	2	2
No decayed teeth	64	34	41	33	36	29	58	20	57	30
No filled† teeth	0	6	0	5	0	16	0	15	0	10
12 or more filled† teeth	54	36	29	27	46	10	74	32	52	29
Natural teeth and dentures	7	11	6	13	18	3	26	18	11	11
Full upper denture	0	0	0	3	0	0	0	3	0	1
BASES	44	47	17	40	11	31	19	40	105	172

Base numbers re-weighted.

*Includes the student, unemployed and unclassifiable categories which are not included elsewhere in the table.
†Filled, otherwise sound.

The youngest age group, that is those aged 16–34 (Table 5.24) is first considered. Having already seen how the dental condition is related to social class and dental attendance pattern, the position in Table 5.24 is much as would be expected. Among those aged 16–34, the regular attenders in the top social class group had a particularly small number of decayed teeth, a large number of filled teeth, and average numbers of sound and untreated teeth. The irregular attenders in the lowest social class group had the highest number of decayed teeth, a low number of filled teeth and a high number of sound and untreated teeth.

Among those aged 35–54 (Table 5.25) social class had some effect both for the regular attenders and the irregular attenders. The regular attenders in the top social class group had 13.3 filled teeth compared to 10.0 among the regular attenders of the lowest social class group; and the irregular attenders in the top social class group had 8.2 filled teeth compared to 5.0 among the irregular attenders in the intermediate social class group.

TABLE 5.25

The Number of Teeth in the Different Conditions for Different Social Classes and Attendance Patterns

Average number of teeth which were:	Adults aged 35–54 with some natural teeth									
	Household Social Class								All* Social Classes	
	I, II and III non-manual		III manual		IV non-manual, IV manual and V		Housewife			
	Regular	Irregular	Regular	Irregular	Regular	Irregular	Regular	Irregular	Regular	Irregular
Missing　.　.　.	8.4	11.2	10.3	12.4	12.0	13.8	9.3	17.1	9.4	12.9
Present　.　.　.	23.6	20.8	21.7	19.6	20.0	18.2	22.7	14.9	22.6	19.1
Decayed　.　.　.	0.7	1.2	1.3	2.1	1.3	2.4	0.8	1.8	0.9	1.9
Filled†　.　.　.	13.3	8.2	10.2	5.9	10.0	5.0	12.7	4.0	12.1	6.0
Sound and untreated .　.	9.1	11.2	10.0	11.5	7.8	10.7	8.9	9.0	9.1	11.0
Teeth at risk　.　.　.	23.1	20.6	21.5	19.5	19.1	18.1	22.4	14.8	22.1	18.9
	%	%	%	%	%	%	%	%	%	%
Proportion of people with:										
18 or more missing teeth	10	12	13	19	18	29	14	50	12	23
No decayed teeth　.　.	62	49	50	31	46	33	52	17	55	35
No filled† teeth　.　.	0	18	0	22	0	13	0	42	0	23
12 or more filled† teeth .	62	36	31	14	45	4	57	8	53	17
Natural teeth and dentures .	21	36	38	42	27	46	38	58	31	44
Full upper denture　.　.	8	9	6	6	9	22	5	42	7	14
BASES　.　.　.	42	33	16	36	11	24	21	12	93	110

*Includes the student, unemployed and unclassifiable categories which are not included in the table.
†Filled, otherwise sound.

It is always of value, when there are two (or more) factors, each of which appear to be of importance, to compare their relative importance. Considerable social class differences, dental attendance pattern differences and differences in the condition of the natural teeth were found.

6. The Gum Condition of Dentate Adults

One of the main causes of tooth loss is poor oral hygiene resulting in decay and gum disease. Poor oral hygiene can result from irregularities of the teeth and gums as well as from neglect. For this reason attention was paid to debris, calculus, gingivitis and periodontal involvement.

6.1 Conditions which Affect the Health of the Gums

(a) DEBRIS

The debris measurement was taken at 6 segments in the mouth, three in the upper jaw and three in the lower, left, middle and right.

The dentist examined these segments in accordance with the criteria (Appendix 5) and scored the segment 0 or 1 as follows:—

0—No soft deposits.

1—Soft deposits clearly visible to the unaided eye at the gingival margin of one or more of the teeth.

Overall, 89% of segments were debris free with some variation between segments. In particular, the lower anterior segment had appreciably more debris than the other segments while the upper anterior segment had less than the other segments.

A much higher proportion of upper jaw segments were unassessed because of missing teeth than were lower jaw segments.

TABLE 6.1

Debris per Segment, among Adults, of All Ages, with Some Natural Teeth

Debris	Adults with some natural teeth						
	Segment						All Segments
	UL	UM	UR	LR	LM	LL	
	%	%	%	%	%	%	%
0	87	90	87	90	87	91	89
1	8	5	8	8	12	7	8
No assessment*	5	5	5	2	1	2	3
	100	100	100	100	100	100	100
BASES	592	592	592	592	592	592	3,552

*All teeth missing in particular segment.

TABLE 6.2

Total Debris Score (Sum of all Segments) for Adults, of All Ages, with Some Natural Teeth

Total debris score	Adults with some natural teeth
	%
Zero	79
One or Two	14
Three or Four	5
Five or Six	2
	100
BASE	592

26

(b) CALCULUS

The basis of the calculus assessment was similar to the debris assessment. The same six segments were used three in the upper jaw and three in the lower.

Again the dentist scored the locations on a scale 0, 1 as follows:—

0—No calculus or deposits not calcified.

1—Calculus in contact with the gingival margin of one or more teeth with a segment. Obvious deposits suspected of being calcified on unaided eye inspection or with the aid of a mirror were tested with a periodontal probe to ensure that they were in fact calcified.

Only 80% of segments were calculus free compared to 89% which were debris free. As Table 6.3 shows the lower anterior segment was approximately five times more prone to calculus than any other segment.

TABLE 6.3

Calculus Score per Segment for Adults, of All Ages, with Some Natural Teeth

Calculus	Adults with some natural teeth						
	Segment						All Segments
	UL	UM	UR	LR	LM	LL	
Score:	%	%	%	%	%	%	%
0	85	90	88	85	43	87	80
1	10	5	7	12	56	11	17
No assessment* . . .	5	5	5	2	1	2	3
	100	100	100	100	100	100	100
BASES	592	592	592	592	592	592	3,552

*All teeth missing in particular segment.

While a high proportion of segments were calculus free (80%) only 42% of adults were free of calculus in all locations. A higher proportion (46%) evidenced calculus in either one or two segments.

TABLE 6.4

Total Calculus Score (Sum of all Segments) for Adults, of All Ages, with Some Natural Teeth

Total Calculus score	Adults with some natural teeth
	%
Zero	42
One or Two	46
Three or Four	10
Five or Six	2
	100
BASE	592

(c) GINGIVITIS

The debris and calculus indicators were assessed in six chosen segments. The same segments were used to assess the degree of inflammation in the gingivae. Scores of 0, 1 and 2 were used as follows:—

0—Gums are not inflamed, pale pink, healthy and firm. No treatment is indicated.

1—Moderate gingivitis. The gingival margin is reddish and slightly oedematous. There is a tendency to bleed. The gingivitis should respond to plaque control alone.

2—Intense gingivitis. The gingivae are markedly red, oedematous and bleed on digital pressure.

TABLE 6.5

Gingivitis Score per Segment for Adults, of All Ages, with Some Natural Teeth

| Gingivitis Score | Adults with some natural teeth | | | | | | |
| | Segment | | | | | | All Segments |
	UL	UM	UR	LR	LM	LL	
	%	%	%	%	%	%	%
0	83	81	83	85	75	85	82
1	11	13	11	11	19	11	13
2	1	1	1	2	5	1	2
No assessment*	5	5	5	2	1	3	3
	100	100	100	100	100	100	100
BASES	592	592	592	592	592	592	3,552

*All teeth missing in particular segment.

Although 82% of segments were free from inflammation, the lower middle segment was clearly more prone to gingivitis with only 75% of these segments gingivitis free.

Overall, 67% of dentate adults managed to keep all their teeth free from inflammation, 17% having a summed score of one or two with a similar proportion having more extreme scores, (Table 6.6).

TABLE 6.6

Total Gingivitis Score (Sum of All Segments) for Adults, of All Ages, with Some Natural Teeth

Total Gingivitis score	Adults with some natural teeth
	%
Zero	67
One or two	17
Three or four	9
Five or six	5
More than six	2
	100
BASE	592

(d) PERIODONTAL INVOLVEMENT

Diseases involving the periodontal tissues are of considerable interest in a study of adult dental health. Periodontal disease is regarded as a more likely cause of tooth loss among adults than dental decay. The destruction of the periodontal attachment, inflammation and pocket formation were all investigated during the survey. Appendix 5 shows the method of classifying periodontal conditions. The classification was the same as that used in the 1978 UK Adult Dental Health Survey.

The six segments used to locate deposits, calculus and gingivitis were also used to locate periodontitis. The classification used was:—

0—No periodontitis is present.
1—Periodontitis is present.

TABLE 6.7

Total Periodontitis Score (Sum of All Segments) for Adults, of All Ages, with Some Natural Teeth

Total Periodontitis score	Adults with some natural teeth
	%
Zero	86
One or two	11
Three or four	2
Five or six	1
	100
BASE	592

In all 14% of the sample showed signs of periodontitis but only 3% had total scores of three or more.

TABLE 6.8

Periodontitis Score per Segment for Adults, of All Ages, with Some Natural Teeth

Periodontitis score	Adults with some natural teeth						
	Segment						All Segments
	UL	UM	UR	LR	LM	LL	
	%	%	%	%	%	%	%
0	92	90	92	94	89	93	92
1	3	5	3	4	10	4	5
No assessment* . . .	5	5	5	2	1	3	3
	100	100	100	100	100	100	100
BASES	592	592	592	592	592	592	3,552

*All teeth missing in particular segment.

(e) CROWDING

A factor which can contribute to the health or disease of the gum tissues is crowding. The natural stimulation of the gums which comes about through chewing, speech or cheek and tongue movements can be impaired by the crowding of the teeth. Cleaning by toothbrushing, sticks or floss can be difficult. The greater the degree of crowding, the greater may be the effect on the gums. Food stasis, build up of debris and plaque and gingival hyperplasia can all result from crowding. Crowding was evaluated in the six segments.

The range of scores for crowding was as follows:—

0—No crowding, the standing teeth fit into the segment without overlapping or irregularity.

1—Shortage of space in the segment to the extent of not more than one lower lateral incisor width (lower middle segment) one upper lateral incisor width (upper middle segment) or one premolar width (left and right segments).

2—There is a shortage of space, an overlap or irregularity to a greater extent than in the range of score 1.

TABLE 6.9

Total Crowding Score (Sum of All Segments) for Adults, of All Ages, with Some Natural Teeth

Total Crowding score	Adults with some natural teeth
	%
Zero	90
One or two	9
Three to six	1
	100
BASE	592

(f) OVERJET AND OVERBITE

Because they have a bearing on dental health, speech, mastication and appearance, overjet and overbite are of interest in dental health surveys. The overjet is the amount by which the upper teeth project over the lower teeth. This relationship can be measured. For the purposes of the survey the measurement of the overjet was recorded in millimetres. In an edge to edge bite no measurement is possible. The lower teeth can project in front of the upper teeth resulting in a reverse overjet. In such cases the overjet was recorded as negative and the overjet recorded in millimetres in the ordinary way. The criteria are recorded in Appendix 5.

The overbite is the relationship between the upper and lower incisor teeth. In the normal occlusion the upper incisor teeth overlap the lower incisor teeth by about one third of the length of the crown of the lower incisors. The assessment of overbite and overjet was made only where there was sufficient posterior support to maintain consistent occlusion and where natural incisor teeth were present.

TABLE 6.10

Overbite and Overjet for Adults with Incisor Teeth

Overjet	%	Overbite	%
Positive	90	1. (No overlap)	14
Negative	3	2. (Overlap less than $1/3$) . . .	47
Zero	7	3. (Overlap more than $1/3$) . . .	39
	100		100

29

6.2 The Gum Condition of Dentate Adults by Age, Sex and Social Class

Table 6.11 shows that the proportion of dentate adults who had no debris did not vary with age, about four out of five adults in each age group being debris-free.

There was a considerable decline with age in the proportion of dentate adults who were calculus-free. Among those aged 16–24, 62% were calculus-free, but among those who were 55 and over only 32% were calculus-free. As with debris, the proportion of people with some calculus present increased over the age groups. 38% of those aged 16–24 had calculus compared with 60% among those aged 25–34, 70% among those aged 35–44, 65% among those aged 45–54 and 68% among those aged 55 and over. This was a considerable increase when one remembers that in middle and older age groups more people have become edentulous and thus been excluded, leaving, presumably, the more dentally fit.

The gingivitis score demonstrated that 67% of persons with some natural teeth were free of gingivitis.

In terms of periodontal health 86% of people with some natural teeth were completely free from trouble. Among the younger age groups periodontal disease was fairly uncommon, only 7% of those aged 16–24 and 10% aged 25–34 having a periodontal condition compared with 37% of the 55 year old plus subjects.

In general more women were free of debris, calculus, gingivitis and periodontitis than men. Where debris or calculus were present the tendency was for a higher percentage of men than women to be included in the sample. A similar situation was found for gingivitis and periodontitis (Table 6.12).

The results were examined to see if there was any association between gum condition and social class (Table 6.13). Three divisions of social class plus that of housewives were used.

The proportion of people free from debris was fairly constant over the groups. The proportion of people with some debris increased from 16% to 28% between the top and lowest social class groups.

There was also a tendency towards an increase in the proportion of persons with calculus, gingivitis and periodontitis between the top and the lowest social class groups.

As has been shown there was a variation with age (Table 6.11). A summary of the gum conditions both for social class and for different age groups for debris, calculus, and periodontal trouble is shown in Table 6.14.

TABLE 6.11

Oral Hygiene and Gum Condition in Adults of Different Ages

	Adults with some natural teeth					
	Present Age					All Ages
	16–24	25–34	35–44	45–54	55 and Over	
DEBRIS	%	%	%	%	%	%
Debris free . .	79	83	77	81	72	79
Debris present . .	21	17	23	19	28	21
	100	100	100	100	100	100
CALCULUS	%	%	%	%	%	%
Calculus free . . .	62	40	30	35	32	42
Calculus present . .	38	60	70	65	68	58
	100	100	100	100	100	100
GINGIVITIS	%	%	%	%	%	
Gingivitis free . .	75	71	62	69	51	67
Moderate gingivitis only	18	23	31	29	39	27
Intense gingivitis . .	7	6	7	2	10	6
	100	100	100	100	100	100
PERIODONTAL DISEASE	%	%	%	%	%	%
Periodontal disease free	93	90	89	88	63	86
Periodontitis present .	7	10	11	12	37	14
	100	100	100	100	100	100

TABLE 6.12

Oral Hygiene and Gum Condition in Adults of Different Ages and Sexes

	Adults with some natural teeth											
	Present Age										All Ages	
	16–24		25–34		35–44		45–54		55 and over			
	M	F	M	F	M	F	M	F	M	F	M	F
DEBRIS	%	%	%	%	%	%	%	%	%	%	%	%
Debris free . . .	70	87	81	84	67	85	78	85	62	81	72	85
Debris present . .	30	13	19	15	33	15	22	15	38	19	28	15
	100	100	100	100	100	100	100	100	100	100	100	100
CALCULUS												
Calculus free . . .	56	67	36	43	22	37	30	40	24	40	35	47
Calculus present . .	44	33	64	57	78	63	70	60	76	60	65	53
	100	100	100	100	100	100	100	100	100	100	100	100
GINGIVITIS												
Gingivitis free . .	67	82	70	71	60	64	67	70	51	50	64	59
Moderate gingivitis only	25	13	24	23	31	31	29	30	38	40	28	26
Intense gingivitis . .	8	5	6	6	9	5	4	0	11	10	8	5
	100	100	100	100	100	100	100	100	100	100	100	100
PERIODONTAL DISEASE												
Periodontal disease free .	88	96	90	90	84	92	87	90	62	65	83	88
Periodontal disease present	12	4	10	10	16	8	13	10	38	35	17	12
	100	100	100	100	100	100	100	100	100	100	100	100

TABLE 6.13

Oral Hygiene and Gum Condition for Different Social Class Groups of Adults

	Adults with some natural teeth				
	Household Social Class				All Social Classes
	I, II and III non-manual	III manual	IV non-manual, IV manual and V	Housewife	
DEBRIS	%	%	%	%	%
Debris free	84	74	72	82	79
Debris present . . .	16	26	28	18	21
	100	100	100	100	100
CALCULUS					
Calculus free . . .	48	34	34	45	42
Calculus present . .	52	66	66	55	58
	100	100	100	100	100
GINGIVITIS					
Gingivitis free . . .	72	62	65	64	67
Moderate gingivitis only .	23	31	27	29	27
Intense gingivitis . . .	5	7	8	7	6
	100	100	100	100	100
PERIODONTAL DISEASE					
Periodontal disease free .	91	83	84	86	86
Periodontal disease present .	9	17	16	14	14
	100	100	100	100	100

TABLE 6.14

Summary of Oral Hygiene and Gum Conditions for Different Ages and Social Classes

| | Adults with some natural teeth | | | | | |
| | Present Age | | | | | All Ages |
	16–24	25–34	35–44	45–54	55 and over	
Proportion debris free	%	%	%	%	%	%
SCI, II, III non-manual	82	86	84	89	75	84
SCIII manual	75	87	65	76	65	74
SCIV, V	74	80	50	64	75	72
Housewife	80	79	90	100	79	82
ALL*	79	83	77	81	72	79
Proportion calculus free						
SCI, II, III non-manual	63	40	30	46	46	48
SCIII manual	71	33	23	14	20	34
SCIV, V	37	32	25	36	33	34
Housewife	75	45	38	45	29	45
ALL*	62	40	30	35	32	42
Proportion gingivitis free						
SCI, II, III non-manual	73	70	72	76	64	72
SCIII manual	71	73	58	71	30	62
SCIV, V	74	72	36	57	75	65
Housewife	80	67	62	73	46	64
ALL*	75	71	62	69	51	67
Proportion periodontal disease free						
SCI, II, III non-manual	93	93	91	97	71	91
SCIII manual	89	90	87	90	50	83
SCIV, V	95	88	64	71	67	84
Housewife	100	88	95	91	63	86
ALL*	93	90	89	88	63	86
BASE NUMBERS						
SCI, II, III non-manual	54	42	42	35	27	200
SCIII manual	28	30	31	21	20	130
SCIV, V	19	25	21	14	12	98
Housewife	20	42	22	11	24	119
ALL*	148	143	122	86	93	592

*Includes those not in above categories.

6.3 The Gum Condition of Dentate Adults by Dental Attendance Pattern

In the discussion of the relationship between decay and its treatment and dental attendance, it was shown that the overall condition of the natural teeth was related to attendance pattern. Persons who chose to go to the dentist for a regular check-up had more evidence of restorative dental treatment than irregular attenders. In this section a similar relationship between gum condition and dental attendance pattern is investigated.

Several aspects of the gum condition may be related to dental attendance, debris is the first considered. Soft debris consists of bacteria and food deposits around the teeth and can build up over a short period of time, days rather than weeks. The extent of debris could be expected to be less directly related to attendance pattern and more related to other factors, in particular the frequency of tooth brushing (Chapter 13). Calculus, on the other hand is probably more affected by intervention by the dentist, since once calculus has built up on the teeth it can only be removed professionally. Those people who attend the dentist regularly do, of course, have a much greater opportunity to have any calculus removed, by having a "scale and polish" and therefore the calculus indicator could be expected to be associated with the dental attendance pattern. The relationship between periodontal involvement and dental attendance may be less straightforward, since it is likely that attendance pattern and personal dental habits both play a role. For example, adequate tooth brushing can probably reduce the amount of inflammation.

As Table 6.15 shows, the regular attenders have a higher percentage of persons free from debris, calculus, gingivitis and periodontitis than the non-regular attenders. It is probable that the regular attenders are those with a real interest in their own oral health, active in the pursuit and maintenance of it and are therefore a select and highly motivated group.

It should be remembered also that the standards of debris, calculus, gingivitis and periodontitis recorded in the tables in this Chapter result from a dental examination. The dental examiners were required to take a detached view of the informants dental health and had been trained to record conditions to defined standards and criteria. Further investigation of possible links between regular dental attendance, frequent toothbrushing and the health of the gums and oral tissues could prove to be of interest.

Whether the person goes to the dentist for a regular check-up or not, those who visit the dentist even occasionally are more likely to be encouraged to look after their gums than the non-attenders. They may have a greater chance of having any serious periodontal conditions rectified.

Table 6.15 gives the condition of the gums for the different attendance patterns, and each aspect of the gum condition is examined in turn. In terms of debris there was some variation with dental attendance, in that debris was somewhat more common among those who only went to the dentist when having trouble. 87% of the regular attenders were debris-free compared to 75% of the occasional attenders and 74% of the irregular attenders.

As expected, there was more variation with dental attendance in the case of calculus. The proportions calculus-free were 56%, 33% and 33% over the three attendance groups.

The regular attenders had a higher proportion free of gingivitis (75%) than either the occasional attenders (74%) or those who visited the dentist only when having trouble (58%).

The regular dental attenders again had the highest number free of periodonitis. Nine out of ten (93%) of the regular attenders had no periodontal involvement, compared to 92% of the occasional attenders and 80% of the irregular attenders.

TABLE 6.15

Oral Hygiene and Gum Condition for Different Attendance Patterns

	Adults with some natural teeth			
	Regular check-up	Occasional check-up	Only when having trouble	All
DEBRIS	%	%	%	%
Debris free	87	75	74	79
Debris present	13	25	26	21
CALCULUS				
Calculus free	56	33	33	42
Calculus present	44	67	67	58
GINGIVITIS				
Gingivitis free	75	74	58	67
Moderate gingivitis only	23	19	32	27
Intense gingivitis	2	7	10	6
PERIODONTITIS				
Periodontitis free	93	92	80	86
Periodontitis present	7	8	20	14
BASE	234	73	285	592

Attendance pattern is, therefore, of considerable importance in relation to the condition of the gums, but the relationship is not necessarily a direct one resulting from the actual attendance at the dentist. It is likely that other factors which determine attendance pattern, such as dental awareness and general attitudes towards oral hygiene, also affect personal habits which determine the condition of the gums. In circumstances where overall attitudes are affecting both personal habits (such as tooth cleaning) and dental attendance pattern it is very difficult to disentangle the direct relationship of tooth cleaning with dental health and dental attendance with dental health. A more detailed examination of tooth cleaning will be found in Chapter 13.

It appears that the condition of the gums is related to social class, the higher social classes having a better gum condition on the whole than the lower social classes. It is of value to look at the condition of the gums in relation to social class and attendance pattern to see if these two variables are acting independently and, if so, which seems to be the more important in determining gum condition. If social class and dental attendance are indeed acting independently then the best gum conditions should exist among the regular attenders in the top social class group, and the worst among the irregular attenders of the lowest social class group. This is in fact the case, as is seen in Table 6.16. The table gives the proportion of people who were free of debris, calculus, gingivitis and periodontitis by different social classes and attendance patterns.

In this Chapter the overall gum condition of adults and the variation of gum condition according to age, sex, social class and dental attendance pattern has been discussed. A summary of oral hygiene and gum conditions by attendance pattern and social class is shown in Table 6.16.

Regular dental attenders were found to have healthier gum conditions than irregular attenders, although this relationship may have been influenced more by the attitudes which led to the attendance pattern than to any direct intervention by the dentist.

Improvements in dental health in terms of both decay (and its treatment) and gum condition seem to depend upon attitudes to dentistry and oral hygiene.

TABLE 6.16

Summary of Oral Hygiene and Gum Conditions by Attendance Pattern and Social Class

	Adults with some natural teeth			
	Regular Check-up	Occasional Check-up	Only when having trouble	All
Proportion debris free	%	%	%	%
SCI, II, III non-manual	89	83	77	84
SCIII manual	77	76	72	74
SCIV, V	88	47	72	72
Housewife	87	93	75	82
ALL*	87	75	74	79
Proportion calculus free				
SCI, II, III non-manual	56	30	37	48
SCIII manual	49	24	29	34
SCIV, V	50	27	30	34
Housewife	57	50	34	45
ALL*	56	33	33	42
Proportion gingivitis free				
SCI, II, III non-manual	77	74	64	72
SCIII manual	69	82	55	62
SCIV, V	85	47	60	65
Housewife	66	86	55	64
ALL*	75	74	58	67
Proportion periodontitis free				
SCI, II, III non-manual	94	87	88	91
SCIII manual	86	94	79	83
SCIV, V	96	87	77	84
Housewife	91	100	77	86
ALL*	93	92	80	86
BASE NUMBERS				
SCI, II, III non-manual	102	22	76	200
SCIII manual	35	17	78	130
SCIV, V	27	15	49	98
Housewife	48	14	57	119
ALL*	234	73	285	592

*Includes the student, unemployed and unclassifiable categories which are not included elsewhere in the table.

6.4 The State of the Gums

Persons with some natural teeth of their own were asked about the condition of their gums. 3% said that their gums were swollen at the time of the interview, 4% said that their gums were redder than usual and 18% said that their gums bled, for example when the teeth were brushed.

15% of persons had been given advice on the care of the gums, 86% of those advised by the dentist, 14% by a dental nurse of hygienist. The majority were given general advice on gum care.

7. The Provision of Dentures in Conjunction with the Natural Teeth

Although some people make the change from natural teeth to full dentures in one step, many people pass through a transitional stage where their remaining natural teeth are augmented by the provision of dentures. These dentures vary very widely in the numbers of teeth they replace, ranging from a single tooth to a full upper and partial lower denture.

7.1 The Range of Natural Tooth Replacement by Dentures

Among adults in Northern Ireland a considerable proportion (20% with partial and 53% if partial and full dentures are included) had been fitted with a denture of some kind, and in Table 7.1 we show the range of replacement that had taken place.

TABLE 7.1

The Range of Replacement by Dentures among the Partially Dentured

Denture pattern	All adults	All dentate adults	Dentate adults with dentures
	%	%	%
No dentures	47	70	0
Full upper, partial lower . . .	2	3.5	12
Full upper, no lower	4	6	19
Partial upper, partial lower . . .	3	4	13
Partial upper, no lower	10	15	51
Partial upper, full lower	0.3	0.5	1.5
No upper, partial lower . . .	0.7	1	3
No upper, full lower			0.5
No natural teeth	33	0	0
	100	100	100
BASES	1,176	783	233

Base numbers re-weighted.

Table 7.1 shows that among adults who had dentures in conjunction with natural teeth, 96.5%* had an upper denture of some sort, whereas only 30%† had a lower denture. By far the most common situation was a partial upper denture and no lower denture. A high proportion, (31%) of partially-dentured people had a full denture in the upper jaw, that is 9.5% of all dentate adults had a full upper denture.

Chapter 5 showed that the level of tooth loss among those with some natural teeth varied with age, sex and social class, and therefore the provision of dentures could be expected to vary with these factors also. The range of replacement for adults of different ages, sexes and social classes is given in Tables 7.2–7.4. While the main part of each table shows the variation in the range of provision for those with dentures (ie the 233 people shown in Table 7.1), at the foot of each table the overall proportion of dentate adults who have dentures is also given.

---

*All groups shown in Table 7.1 which included an upper denture.
†All groups shown in Table 7.1 which included a lower denture.

TABLE 7.2

The Range of Replacement by Dentures for Adults of Different Ages

Denture pattern	Adults with some natural teeth who have a denture					
	16–24	25–34	Present age 35–44	45–54	55 and over	All ages
	%	%	%	%	%	%
Full upper, partial lower	0	6	10	10	19	12
Full upper, no lower	0	6	26	16	23	19
Partial upper, partial lower	0	14	14	12	14	13
Partial upper, no lower	100	66	50	56	36	51
Partial upper, full lower	0	3	0	2	3	1.5
No upper, partial lower	0	5	0	4	4	3
No upper, full lower	0	0	0	0	1	0.5
	100	100	100	100	100	100
BASES—dentate adults who have a denture	8	35	62	50	78	233
Proportion of all dentate adults who have a denture	% 4	% 19	% 38	% 41	% 59	% 30
Base numbers re-weighted	182	186	162	121	132	783

As would be expected, the overall proportion of dentate adults who had been fitted with a denture increased steadily with age, from 4% among those aged 16–24, to 59% among those aged 55 and over. Amongst all but the oldest age group the most common denture situation was a partial denture in the upper jaw and no denture in the lower. Among the oldest age group the level of replacement increases, the most common replacement being full denture in the upper jaw. There are, however, considerable numbers of denture wearers who have a full upper denture even among the younger adults. The proportions of denture wearers having a full upper denture are 12, 36 and 26 respectively in the 25–34, 35–44, 45–54 age groups. It is interesting that the proportion of partially-dentured people who have a full upper denture opposing only natural teeth in the lower jaw never falls below the proportion for whom the full upper denture opposes a partial denture in the lower jaw.

In Chapters 4 and 5 there were indications of higher levels of tooth loss among women. The denture pattern for men and women separately is now examined. Table 7.3 shows that among adults with some natural teeth proportionately more women have been fitted with a denture than men (31% compared to 28%). In terms of denture pattern the differences between the sexes are that slightly fewer women have a partial upper denture only, and more have a full upper denture only.

TABLE 7.3

The Range of Replacement by Dentures for Adults of Different Ages and Sexes

Denture pattern	Adults with some natural teeth who have a denture							
	Present age						All ages	
	16–34		35–54		55 and over			
	M	F	M	F	M	F	M	F
	%	%	%	%	%	%	%	%
Full upper, partial lower	6	4	7	12	15	22	10	14
Full upper, no lower	6	4	13	29	27	20	16	21
Partial upper, partial lower	16	8	13	14	12	16	13	13
Partial upper, no lower	72	72	63	43	33	38	55	47
Partial upper, full lower	0	4	0	2	7	0	2	2
No upper, partial lower	0	8	4	0	3	4	3	3
No upper, full lower	0	0	0	0	3	0	1	0
	100	100	100	100	100	100	100	100
BASES—dentate adults who have a denture	18	25	54	58	33	45	105	128
Proportion of all dentate adults who have a denture	% 10	% 13	% 39	% 39	% 56	% 68	% 28	% 31

Base numbers re-weighted.

In the age group 35–54, 41% of dentate women who had been fitted with dentures had a full upper jaw clearance; this compares with 20% for men. For those aged 55 and over, it would appear that by this age men and women are in a similar position with respect to full upper dentures (the proportion with a full upper denture is 42% both for men and women).

We next look, in Table 7.4, at the relative positions of the different social classes with respect to denture pattern. We have found earlier in the report that there were quite considerable social class differences in total tooth loss and in the condition of the natural teeth. Differences occur also in the wearing of dentures. Classes IV and V are more likely to wear full upper dentures than classes I, II and III, whether or not the denture is opposed by natural or artificial teeth. They are also more likely to wear partial upper and lower dentures.

Even in the top social class group, where we might have expected to find less replacement by dentures, just under one quarter of those with some natural teeth have a denture, and for 24% of these denture wearers there is a full clearance of the upper jaw.

TABLE 7.4

The Range of Replacement by Dentures for Different Social Classes

| Denture pattern | Adults with some natural teeth who have a denture | | | | |
| | Household Social Class | | | | |
	I, II and III non-manual	III manual	IV non-manual, IV manual and V	Housewife	All* Social classes
	%	%	%	%	%
Full upper, partial lower	7	10	18	16	12
Full upper, no lower	17	17	24	18	19
Partial upper, partial lower . . .	12	14	18	13	13
Partial upper, no lower	58	54	40	44	51
Partial upper, full lower	1	3	0	2	1.5
No upper, partial lower	5	0	0	7	3
No upper, full lower	0	2	0	0	0.5
	100	100	100	100	100
BASES—dentate adults who have a denture	60	59	38	55	233
Proportion of all dentate adults who have a denture	% 23	% 32	% 29	% 38	% 30

Base numbers re-weighted.

*Includes student, unemployed and unclassifiable categories which are not included elsewhere in the table.

7.2 The Examination Assessment of Dentures

Among dentate adults who had been fitted with dentures and agreed to have an examination, the vast majority (84%) of upper dentures were available for examination, and 82% of lower dentures were available.

In the following tables, as well as giving the situation separately for upper and lower dentures the results are recorded separately whether the upper denture was a full upper denture (replacing 14 teeth) or a partial upper denture (replacing fewer than 14 teeth). Lower dentures are recorded as one group since virtually all of these were partial dentures.

Among the dentures available for examination the vast majority had a base of plastic. Only 2% of full upper dentures were of metal, but 15% of partial upper dentures and 10% of partial lower dentures had a metal base.

Denture hygiene was assessed by the dentist in terms of any debris ie plaque, calculus or stain found on it.

Denture state was assessed either as complete or broken. Dentures were assessed as broken where the denture was fractured, had a missing tooth or had been self-repaired.

Each dental examiner made an assessment of whether the denture required replacement or not.

TABLE 7.5

The Assessment of Denture Hygiene among the Partially-Dentured

Denture material	Upper denture		Lower denture
	Full	Partial	
	%	%	%
Metal	2	15	10
Plastic	98	85	90
	100	100	100
Denture hygiene			
Satisfactory	93	86	83
Not satisfactory	7	14	17
	100	100	100
Denture state			
Complete	93	83	88
Broken	7	17	12
	100	100	100
Replacement of denture required			
Yes	11	18	9
No	89	82	91
	100	100	100
Number of margins			
1–3	0	20	20
4–8	0	60	75
More than 8	100	20	5
	100	100	100
BASES—Dentures available for examination .	45	94	46

Base numbers re-weighted.

Among the partially-dentured a number of dentures were found to be broken at the time of the dental examination (the proportions broken were 7% of full upper dentures, 17% of partial upper dentures and 12% of lower dentures). This level of breakage only reflects the state of those dentures made available for examination, and it is probable that quite a number of the dentures that were not available for examination were damaged.

Table 7.6 shows the mouth conditions found by the examiner among the partially-dentured. Only a condition related to the wearing of partial dentures was assessed, eg gum stripping, tilting and caries on adjacent teeth.

TABLE 7.6

Denture Bearing Areas
The Condition of the Mouth among the Partially Dentured

Condition of mouth	Dentate adults with a denture for the:		
	Upper Jaw		Lower Jaw
	Full	Partial	
	%	%	%
Denture affecting	8	30	33
Not affecting	92	70	67
	100	100	100
BASES	45	94	46

Base numbers re-weighted.

7.3 The Proportion of Dentate Adults who Wear their Dentures

If a person has been provided with dentures then it is in that person's dental interest to wear them, as by not wearing them the person receives less than full dental benefit. All people who said they had not worn their dentures in the four weeks prior to the interview were recorded as non-denture wearers.

TABLE 7.7

The Wearing of Dentures by the Partially-Dentured*

Wearing of dentures	Dentate adults who have a denture
	%
Upper denture only, not worn . . .	9
Lower denture only, not worn . . .	1
One or both dentures not worn† . .	9
Dentures worn, but not all day . . .	6
Dentures worn	75
	100
BASE	233

Base number re-weighted.

†Refers to those having 2 plates so does not include categories 1 or 2.

*Categories relating to dentures worn refer to those available dentures, ie a person with only an upper denture who wears it all day would be included in the same category as a person who has upper and lower dentures and wears them all day. Actual numbers of dentures are not relevant to the last two groups; they refer to the wearing of each individuals total number of plates.

Three quarters (75%) of those people who had been provided with a denture or dentures to complement their natural teeth were in the habit of wearing the denture (Table 7.7). Although, in terms of usage, the majority were receiving some benefit from their dentures, 19% of the partially-dentured had a combination of natural teeth and dentures that was proving unacceptable, since they did not wear one (or both) of their dentures at all. Twice as many upper dentures were said to be lost or broken than lower dentures.

A small proportion of the partially-dentured (6%) wore their dentures some of the time but not all day, and it would thus appear that if a denture proves to be unacceptable then it tends not to be worn at all rather than worn for only part of the time. We asked those who wore their dentures some but not all of the time, to describe when the dentures were and were not worn, and the most common situation for the upper and for the lower was that the denture was worn for appearances only.

Among dentate adults denture wearing varied for different groups of people. There was some variation with age. All of the youngest people wore their dentures all day which was more than other people. Sixty-eight per cent of the oldest age group (55+) wore their dentures all day. A similar proportion of men and women did not wear their dentures at all (20% of men and 18% of women*), but fewer people in the top social class group did not wear them (the proportions not wearing their dentures were 15%, 17% and 21% over the three social class groups). There was an interesting variation with the length of time since the person last visited the dentist, the proportion who did not wear their dentures at all increasing steadily from 12% among those whose visit was in the last 6 months to 42% among those whose last visit was more than 3 years ago.

The dentures provided for dentate adults varied widely. Table 7.8 shows that the extent of wearing is very much related to the denture pattern and looks in detail at each of the denture combinations.

Considered firstly are those people who have lost all of their upper natural teeth and have been fitted with a full upper denture, but still retain some of their natural lower teeth and also have a lower denture. The great majority (60%) were in the habit of wearing their dentures all day. However 36% did not wear one or both at all. Where there is only a full upper denture, and no lower the vast majority (89%) of people wore the upper denture all day.

Next considered are those people who retained some natural teeth in the upper jaw, but who had had some upper teeth replaced by a denture and had no lower denture. Among this group, the majority (80%) wore their partial upper denture all day. Although four out of five were therefore obtaining the maximum benefit, this was not such a high proportion as among people with a full upper denture only. It was, however, a much higher level of wearing than that found among the next group, that is those who had a partial denture in the lower jaw as well as in the upper jaw. Among people who also had a partial lower denture about two thirds (65%) wore both the upper and the lower all the time. This combination of dentures thus appeared to be less acceptable to the wearer.

*Obtained by adding the first three categories together.

TABLE 7.8

The Wearing of Dentures by the Partially-Dentured according to Denture Pattern

	Dentate adults who have a denture			
Wearing of Dentures	Denture pattern			
	Full upper partial lower	*Full upper no lower*	*Partial upper no lower*	*Partial upper partial lower*
Upper only not worn	0	7	14	0
Lower only not worn	0	0	0	0
One or both not worn . . .	36	0	0	32
Dentures worn, but not all day . .	4	4	6	3
Dentures worn all day	60	89	80	65
	100	100	100	100
BASES	28	44	31	118

Base numbers re-weighted.

A small number of people had a pattern of dentures other than those given in Table 7.8, for example a denture in the lower jaw only or a partial upper denture opposing a full lower denture. These patterns also appeared to be somewhat unsatisfactory but the numbers concerned were too small for detailed analysis. It would seem, therefore, that some combinations of dentures are much more acceptable to the wearer than others. An upper denture appeared to be more acceptable than a lower, and a full upper denture was somewhat more acceptable than a partial upper denture.

So far the pattern of dentures in terms of whether they were full or partial dentures and for which jaw they were constructed has been discussed. Next the replacement of some front teeth or some back teeth or both is examined. As can be seen from Tables 7.9 and 7.10 appearance seems to be a contributory factor. Those dentures which involved front tooth replacement were more often worn all day than were the denture replaced back teeth only. Table 7.9 deals with those people whose only denture was a partial upper. If the denture replaced front teeth only, then 78% were worn all day; where the denture involved back teeth only, then 65% were worn all day.

TABLE 7.9

The Wearing of Partial Upper Dentures according to which Teeth Replaced

	Dentate adults who have a denture	
Wearing of partial upper denture	Denture replaces:	
	Some front teeth	*All back teeth*
Denture not worn	17	29
Denture worn, but not all day . . .	5	6
Dentures worn all day	78	65
BASES	124	35

Base numbers re-weighted.
Front = 159   Back = 66 — partials.

Table 7.10 deals with those people whose partial denture was in the lower jaw. Dentures which involved front teeth were more frequently said to be worn all day (76%) than those which involved back teeth only (54%).

TABLE 7.10

The Wearing of Partial Lower Dentures according to which Teeth Replaced

	Dentate adults who have a denture	
Wearing of partial lower denture	Denture replaces:	
	Some front teeth	*Back teeth only*
Denture not worn	16	41
Denture worn, but not all day . . .	8	5
Denture worn all day	76	54
	100	100
BASES	25	46

Base numbers re-weighted.

7.4 Some of the Difficulties of Having Dentures

The importance of appearance in relation to the wearing of dentures and the fact that some types of dentures are less likely to be worn than others has been noted in the report. Sometimes the fit, as assessed by the dentist, had no bearing on whether the denture was worn or not. These findings suggest that the difficulties encountered by people who have dentures, and the personal adjustments which need to be made, will be met by different reactions. Some people will stop wearing their dentures and others will continue wearing them despite the difficulties encountered. During the interview those who had dentures were asked whether certain everyday experiences caused them any difficulties because of their dentures. We included people who were not currently wearing their dentures and asked them whether they had, or would have, experienced any difficulties, since some people may have given up wearing their dentures because of such difficulties.

The results (in Table 7.11) are presented separately for those who wear their dentures and those who do not. The results are recorded separately for each jaw. The everyday circumstances asked about were yawning, talking, chewing meat and biting into a raw apple. We also asked the person whether he felt his dentures were too loose or too tight, and whether they had made his mouth sore at all in the previous four weeks.

In most cases the lower denture caused more difficulties than the upper. Such a result is not unexpected as lower dentures being less well supported by the oral tissues tend to cause more problems than upper dentures. Among people who wore their dentures all day, yawning caused problems in 5% of upper denture wearers and in 12% of lower denture wearers. Talking caused problems for 7% and 12% respectively. People who no longer wore their dentures had experienced difficulties with the lower denture when yawning (25%) and talking (33%) but none with the upper denture.

TABLE 7.11

Difficulties with Dentures among the Partially-Dentured*

Whether person has had difficulties with:		Dentate adults who have a denture					
		Upper denture			Lower denture		
		One of two Not† worn	Worn part of day	Worn all day	One of two Not† worn	Worn part of day	Worn all day
		%	%	%	%	%	%
Yawning	Difficulties	0	0	5	25	0	12
	None	100	100	95	75	100	88
		100	100	100	100	100	100
Talking	Difficulties	0	25	7	33	0	12
	None	100	75	93	67	100	88
		100	100	100	100	100	100
Chewing meat	Difficulties	14	25	10	25	0	16
	None	86	75	90	75	100	84
		100	100	100	100	100	100
Biting into a raw apple	Difficulties	15	100	19	75	50	21
	None	85	0	81	25	50	79
		100	100	100	100	100	100
Fit of dentures	Too loose	14	25	15	50	100	23
	About right	86	75	85	50	0	77
	Too tight	0	0	0	0	0	0
		100	100	100	100	100	100
Comfort of dentures	Hurt	7	25	3	25	50	14
	Not	93	75	93	75	50	86
		100	100	100	100	100	100
BASES		14	4	171	4	2	43

Base numbers re-weighted.

*Asked only of those who had worn the denture in the 4 weeks prior to the interview.

†One of two not worn means the question was asked of those who had 2 dentures but wore only one.

Chewing meat appeared to be somewhat difficult. The upper and lower dentures were both troublesome for those whose dentures were worn all day, the proportion causing trouble were 10% and 16% for the upper and the lower dentures respectively. Those who did not wear one of their dentures had had trouble where chewing meat was concerned, the proportions having difficulties being 14% and 25% for upper and lower dentures respectively.

For people who wear their dentures, biting into a raw apple was the most difficult task for both dentures (the proportions having trouble biting into a raw apple were 19% and 21% for upper and lower dentures respectively). Overall, the people who did not wear their dentures had had more trouble in this respect, 15% of upper dentures and 75% of lower dentures causing trouble.

Among people who wear their dentures all day, none thought that their dentures were too tight, although 15% of upper dentures and 23% of lower dentures were said to be too loose. Among those who did not wear their dentures, however, 14% of upper and 50% of lower were said to be too loose.

Only a small proportion of those who wear their dentures said that the denture had made the mouth sore (3% of upper and 14% of lower) but one quarter (25%) of the people who wear their upper denture for only part of the day had had trouble in this respect.

7.5 Wearing Partial Dentures

The experiences which persons who had lost some natural teeth had had with their partial dentures were thought to be of interest since they could contribute to attitudes to dental health and to attitudes to the wearing of full dentures.

Persons who had been provided with a partial denture or dentures were asked if they still had their top or bottom plate. Those who still had plates were asked why they did not wear them. The replies varied but the two main reasons were:—

1. Informant was not satisfied with the fit or appearance   (35%)*
2. Dentures hurt, were uncomfortable   (29%)*

Persons who no longer had plates were asked what had happened to them. The most common reason was that they had been lost (87%).

Some persons who have been provided with partial dentures do not wear them during the whole daytime. They were asked when they did wear them.

TABLE 7.12

*Occasions when Partial Denture is Worn**

	Top plate %		Bottom plate %	
	Yes	No	Yes	No
Plate worn when going out . . .	71	29	71	29
Plate worn when eating .	21	79	57	43
Plate worn about the house . . .	21	79	29	71
TOTAL	14		7	

Persons who did not wear their partial dentures all the time were asked why they did not do so. The main reasons were:—

1. The dentures hurt   (30%)
2. They spoil the taste of food   (25%)
3. They look bad   (10%)

Some variation was observed in the age at which persons first had a dentured fitted.

*Very few did not actually wear their partial dentures during the whole daytime.

TABLE 7.13

Age at which First Denture Fitted

	Male	Female
	%	%
16–24	28	37
25–34	26	19
35–44	24	19
45–54	15	16
55–64	5	5
65 and over	1	2
Can't remember age	2	2
TOTAL	105	123

Persons who wear dentures can lose other natural teeth resulting in additions to or replacement of a partial denture or the provision of a full denture. Partial denture wearers were asked how many teeth they had lost since their first set of dentures. Twenty-two per cent reported that they had lost no teeth, 39% 1–5 teeth and 20% had lost 6 or more teeth. (19% gave other answers).

The replacement dentures were supplied for a variety of reasons.

TABLE 7.14

Reasons for the Replacement of Dentures*

	Upper denture				Lower denture			
	Male		Female		Male		Female	
	Yes	No/DK	Yes	No/DK	Yes	No/DK	Yes	No/DK
	%	%	%	%	%	%	%	%
More teeth extracted	44	56	41	59	30	70	39	61
Previous denture hurt or caused ulcers . .	4	96	11	89	10	90	6	94
Previous denture worn down, damaged or broken	19	81	48	52	20	80	28	72
Previous denture did not fit properly . .	23	77	22	78	30	70	41	59
Previous denture did not look right . .	8	92	11	89	0	100	0	100
Previous denture did not match the other denture	4	96	0	100	0	100	6	94
Other reasons	8	92	6	94	11	89	0	100

*85 had top plates replaced; 28 had lower plates replaced.

7.6 The Cleansing of Dentures

The dental examination provided an assessment of dental status. This assessment included an evaluation by the dental examiner of denture hygiene. In addition to the examination information, informants were asked about denture hygiene. Twenty per cent found it difficult to clean dentures and 80% found no difficulty. Forty-five per cent cleaned their teeth once per day, 45% twice or more, 10% once per week or less frequently. Forty-five per cent cleansed by soaking, 84% by brushing and 1% by some other method. (Cleaning methods were not mutually exclusive).

A high percentage, 78%, soaked their dentures in powder solutions. Of persons who brushed their dentures 84% brushed them with toothpaste or toothpowder, 10% used a denture cleaner, and 6% used other substances eg soap and water.

7.7 Denture Adhesives and Measures to Relieve Soreness

Among partial denture wearers, the use of denture adhesives could be expected to be uncommon since most partial dentures receive a measure of support from the natural teeth. Of the partial denture wearers interviewed for the survey 6% used a denture adhesive and 94% did not.

Informants who wore partial dentures were asked if they used anything to prevent or ease soreness. One per cent said that they had taken tablets or lozenges and 99% that they had not.

7.8 History of Denture Currently in Use

Persons who were wearing dentures were asked how long ago they had been provided with their denture.

TABLE 7.15

Length of Time since Present Denture was Fitted — Upper Denture

	Male %	Female %
Less than 1 year	8	10
1 year less than 2 years . . .	10	13
2 years less than 5 years . . .	27	22
5 years less than 10 years . . .	29	29
10 years less than 20 years . . .	20	20
20 years or more	6	6

TABLE 7.16

Length of Time since Present Denture was Fitted — Lower Denture

	Male %	Female %
Less than 1 year	17	10
1 year less than 2 years . . .	3	7
2 years less than 5 years . . .	27	28
5 years less than 10 years . . .	27	22
10 years less than 20 years . . .	17	28
20 years or more	9	5

The vast majority of wearers of partial dentures had obtained them through the Health Service (87% upper, 84% lower) but a small proportion had obtained them privately (10% upper, 12% lower). Those who had obtained dentures privately were asked why. The main reasons were:—

1. Dentures obtained privately are better quality   34%
2. Treatment not available under NHS   20%
3. Wanted dentures quickly   17%

Three per cent did not know or had been fitted with the denture before the Health Service began.

7.9 The Appearance of Partial Dentures

Seventy-two per cent of persons wearing partial dentures said that they wore them for appearance compared with 23% who said that they wore them to help with eating, 5% said both. Several of the questions asked at the interview were related to the appearance of the teeth.

Persons who were wearing partial dentures were asked for their opinions of the appearance of the dentures. Eighty-one per cent said that they were very satisfied, 10% that they were fairly satisfied, 5% not very satisfied and 2% not at all satisfied. Two per cent did not have any view on the appearance. Persons who were less than very satisfied were asked what feature of the appearance of their partial denture did not satisfy them. Twenty-six per cent said they did not look like their natural teeth; 26% said their complaint was actually nothing to do with appearance; and 12% said the teeth were too short and they could not be seen properly.

7.10 Dentist's Advice on the Wearing of Partial Dentures

Advice from the dentist can help the new wearer of partial dentures to overcome the initial strangeness of the prosthesis. Wearers of partial dentures were asked what advice had been given to them by the dentist when they first had dentures fitted.

TABLE 7.17

Dentist's Advice on Wearing Partial Dentures

	Adults with some natural teeth					
	Males			Females		
	%	%	%	%	%	%
	Yes	No	Can't remember	Yes	No	Can't remember
Advice on chewing	15	75	10	7	71	22
Advice on biting	15	75	10	9	73	18
Advice on length of time to get used to dentures	33	55	12	17	66	17
Advice on length of time dentures would be expected to last	2	95	3	5	90	5
Advice on cleaning dentures . . .	24	71	5	15	76	9
Advice on wearing dentures at night . .	30	57	13	34	57	9

7.11 Reactions to New Partial Dentures

The majority of denture wearers (61%) were not told how long it would take to get used to wearing dentures. Of those who were told, the most frequent time-span mentioned by dentists was up to one month (59%). Thirty-two per cent of dentists advised that dentures should be worn at night. Few people (27%) would have liked more advice on managing dentures. The proportion of denture wearers who were given a leaflet about wearing dentures was 4%. Eighty-seven per cent were not and 9% could not remember.

The length of time taken to get used to partial dentures varied from—38% less than one week, 44% 1 week–3 months, 11% over 3 months and 10% were still not used to wearing them. The vast majority (70%) took between 0 and 12 weeks to get used to wearing a denture. Most persons (78%) found nothing unexpected about wearing a denture but it was found that all were conscious of the affect in the mouth, (mouth feeling full (39%), taste affected (13%), difficulty speaking (15%), difficulty chewing (7%), sore or bad fit (17%)).

7.12 Eating with New Partial Dentures

Persons who have been fitted with partial dentures can experience differences in their eating habits. Three per cent of partial denture wearers interviewed said that they enjoyed their food more than before they had dentures, 78% about the same and 18% less than before they had them. Four per cent said that they had to change the kind of food they ate and 96% did not. Eighty-eight per cent reported that there was nothing which they could eat with dentures which they had been unable to eat before being fitted with dentures. Eighty-three per cent said that there was nothing which they could eat previously which they could not eat with dentures.

7.13 Effect of Partial Dentures on the Natural Teeth

Twenty per cent of persons wearing partial dentures said that they had trouble with their natural teeth which they felt was connected with having dentures compared with 80% who felt they had not. The main troubles were:—

1. Wears/rubs causing teeth to rot/decay   34%
2. Wears/rubs causing teeth to come out or loosen   32%
3. Wires/clips cause problems   14%

Thirty-nine per cent of partial denture wearers had lost 1–5 teeth since they started to wear partial dentures, 14% between 5 and 11, 5% between 12 and 20 and 2% over 20.

7.14 Advice to Prospective Partial Denture Wearers

Persons wearing partial dentures were asked what advice they would give to others who might have to have a partial denture for the first time. The advice was:—

1. If your teeth are bad don't hesitate to have them out   30%
2. After dentures are fitted, keep them in, persevere   21%
3. Don't know/would not advise   23%

8. The Provision of Full Dentures

In Northern Ireland the provision of full dentures for those who have had a full clearance is nearly universal, 94% of those with no natural teeth having been fitted with full dentures. The 6% (23 people) who said that they had never been fitted with full dentures was made up of 15 who said that they could manage satisfactorily without dentures and had never bothered to get a set, 2 who were waiting for their first full set of dentures, 1 who expressed apprehension of going to the dentist to get a set, 4 who managed with a full upper denture only, and 1 who mentioned expense as a contributory factor.

Thus, once full clearance has been carried out there is virtually no unmet need for the provision of full dentures, although of course, there may be some unmet need in the community for full clearance.

When discussing the situation of dentate adults who had been provided with dentures one of the main points of interest was the range of teeth that had been replaced, since this varied considerably for different people. The range of replacement is not a major problem when discussing full dentures, since the intention is that all natural teeth will have been replaced by a full upper denture and a full lower denture.

8.1 Characteristics of the Wearers of Full Dentures

TABLE 8.1

Age and Sex of the Edentulous

	Males	Females	All
16–34	1	4	5
35–44	11	17	28
45–54	24	32	56
55–64	43	67	110
65–74	61	67	128
75 and over . .	18	48	66
	158	235	393

60% of the edentulous were female compared to 40% male. 49% were 65 years of age or older with the majority (77%) being 55 years of age or older.

TABLE 8.2

Marital Status of the Edentulous

	Males	Females	All
Married	116	121	237
Single	23	28	51
Widowed/Divorced/Separated	19	86	105
	158	235	393

A small proportion (17%) were single while 60% were married.

The average edentulous person would appear to be over 55 years of age and married, with females more likely to be edentulous than males.

As a result of being more likely to be female aged over 55, the largest single category in the classification of occupations was housewife (38%). If manual occupations are grouped together, these accounted for a further 32%.

TABLE 8.3
Social Class of the Edentulous

	%
Non-manual occupations: (Professional, Intermediate/Managerial, Skilled Non-Manual) . .	19
Manual occupations: (Skilled manual, partly skilled, unskilled)	32
Housewives	38
Other: (Student, unemployed, sick, no occupation given)	11

It should be noted that where a person was not currently in work, a description of the last job was requested. This accounts for the lack of a large category of pensioners which the age distribution would suggest.

Having looked at the characteristics of the edentulous it should be worthwhile to look at their overall dental attitudes.

TABLE 8.4
Attendance Patterns of the Edentulous

	%
Regular check-ups	7
Occasional check-ups	8
Only when having trouble	84.75
Never	0.25

Only one edentulous person claimed never to attend a dentist. (For future tables on attendance patterns, 100% will exclude this one person). The vast majority attended a dentist only when they were having trouble with their teeth.

TABLE 8.5
Previous Experience of Restorative Treatment

	%
No previous restorative treatment . . .	59
Previous treatment	41

In keeping with the finding that most edentulous persons had visited the dentist only when having trouble, the majority of edentulous people had never had any fillings or restorative treatment.

Informants were asked when they lost the last of their own teeth, how many had to be taken out altogether.

TABLE 8.6
Number of Last Remaining Teeth Extracted

	%
1–11	42
12–20	30
21 or more	28

Over half of the edentulous had lost 12 or more teeth at the final clearance. When this final extraction took place only 26% had previously had a denture. Of those 26%, the majority had previously had partial upper dentures (See Table 8.21).

Informants were then asked whether the last of their teeth had been extracted together or were taken out over a series of visits. The majority (59%) had been taken out all at once.

As examinations were made of neither the mouth condition of the edentulous nor of their dentures, information was sought on whether or not those with full dentures actually wore them.

8.2 Do Adults with Full Dentures Wear Their Dentures?

Although the vast majority of people who had lost all their natural teeth had been provided with full dentures, this does not necessarily mean that the dentures were worn. The criteria for wearing were based on whether the dentures had been worn in the four weeks prior to the interview. For dentures that had been worn at least some of the time we further asked whether or not the dentures were worn all the daytime, that is from the time the informant got up until he went to bed.

Table 8.7 shows that the great majority (80%) of those who had been provided with a full set of dentures were in the habit of wearing both the upper and lower denture all the time. There was on the other hand a group of considerable size (17%) who did not wear one or other denture at all; this group was made up of 7% who did not wear either denture and 10% who wore only the upper denture. Where one or both dentures were not worn we asked the informant why this was. The most common reasons for full lower dentures not being worn was that they did not fit well, or had a poor appearance and some of them were said to hurt. The most common reason given for not wearing the upper denture was that it did not look right or looked bad. An equal proportion of upper and lower dentures were said to be lost or so severely damaged that they could not be worn. Of those who did not wear one or the other, lost/thrown away was more common than broken, but very few fitted this group.

TABLE 8.7

The Wearing of Dentures by the Fully-Dentured

Wearing of dentures	Adults who have been fitted with a full set of dentures
	%
One or both dentures not worn . . .	17
Both dentures worn, but not all day . .	3
Both dentures worn all day . . .	80
	100

The remaining group, 3%, were in the habit of wearing their dentures for part of the day only, and information was sought on when the dentures were worn and when they were not. There were no differences between upper and lower dentures as to the times at which they were worn. By far the most common situation was a denture only being worn for appearance's sake, for instance when the informant was out or when eating, (three-quarters of dentures worn for part of the day were worn only for appearance). Of those who did not wear their dentures all day, on average 78% wore them only for eating. Within this very small group, the trend was to wear both upper and lower plates when going out, not to wear them when eating, and definitely not to wear them about the house.

The proportion who wore both dentures all day declined steadily with age (Table 8.8), from 89% among those aged 35–44 to 73% among those aged 75 and over. Among people in the age groups 65–74, almost 1 in 4 did not wear one or other denture at all.

TABLE 8.8

The Wearing of Full Dentures, for Adults of Different Ages

Wearing of dentures	Adults who have been fitted with a full set of dentures						
	Present age						
	16–34	35–44	45–54	55–64	65–74	75 and over	All ages
	%	%	%	%	%	%	%
One or both dentures not worn .	20	7	9	13	24	18	17
Both dentures worn, but not all day	0	4	4	2	1	9	3
Both dentures worn all day . .	80	89	87	85	75	73	80
	100	100	100	100	100	100	100
BASES	5	28	54	108	119	55	369

Base numbers re-weighted.

There was some variation with social class (Table 8.9) in that proportionately more people in the top 2 social class groups were in the habit of wearing both dentures all day (this proportion decreased from 87 in group 2 to 79% over the next three groups.

The most striking feature is that denture wearers are much more likely to come from the lower social classes, this group accounting for 75% of edentulous people studied.

TABLE 8.9

The Wearing of Full Dentures, for Adults of Different Social Classes

Wearing of dentures	Adults who have been fitted with a full set of dentures				
	Household Social Class				
	I, II and III non-manual	III manual	IV non-manual, IV manual, and V	Housewife	All* Social Classes
	%	%	%	%	%
One or both dentures not worn . . .	13	13	18	17	17
Both dentures worn, but not all day . .	4	0	4	3	3
Both dentures worn all day	83	87	78	80	80
	100	100	100	100	100
BASES	52	39	81	138	369

Base numbers re-weighted.
*Includes the student, unemployed and unclassifiable categories which are not included elsewhere in the table.

A difference of habit in the wearing of full dentures was found among women as compared with men. While the vast majority of both sexes wore their full dentures all day, slightly more women (83%) than men (78%) did so.

TABLE 8.10

The Wearing of Full Dentures for Adults according to Length of Time Since Last Extraction

Wearing of dentures	Adults who have been fitted with a full set of dentures						
	Length of time since last natural tooth extracted						
	Up to 5 years	5–10 years	10–15 years	15–20 years	20–30 years	Over 30 years	Total
	%	%	%	%	%	%	%
One or both dentures not worn .	20	20	6	10	21	21	17
Both dentures worn, not all day .	0	2	3	5	3	1	3
Both dentures worn all day .	80	78	90	85	76	78	80
BASES	20	46	68	59	103	71	367*

*Two people could not remember.

Those least likely to wear full dentures all day were those who had had the last of their natural teeth out over 20 years ago. The general picture would appear to be that those who have been edentulous a long time and those who have relatively recently lost the last of their teeth are least likely to wear their full dentures all day.

The vast majority of edentulous (91%) had not visited a dentist within the last year. When asked how long it had actually been since they had last visited the dentist 57% stated they had not been in the last 10 years. The group who had not seen a dentist for 15 years or more were the least likely to wear both plates all day, 26% falling into this category.

8.3 Some of the Difficulties of Wearing Full Dentures

Dentures are rarely a perfect substitute for natural teeth, and can cause the wearer various problems. A proportion of people who had been fitted with dentures were not in fact wearing them at all.

In the interview people with dentures were asked about some everyday situations to see how many of them had difficulties, the everyday situations being yawning, talking, chewing meat and biting into a raw apple. The survey also asked whether full denture wearers thought their dentures were too loose, about right, or too tight, and whether or not the dentures had hurt or made their mouths sore in the four weeks prior to the interview.

Yawning and talking caused problems in similar proportions of cases, but in each of these situations it was the lower denture which was the most troublesome. Of those dentures worn all day, yawning caused problems in 4% and 7% of cases for upper and lower dentures respectively, the proportions for talking being 5% and 8%.

Chewing meat caused rather more problems and again it was the lower denture which was the less satisfactory; of those dentures worn all day, chewing meat caused problems in 8% and 13% of cases for upper and lower dentures respectively.

TABLE 8.11

Difficulties with Full Dentures

This table refers only to those with full dentures who wear them all day

	Adults who have been fitted with a full set of dentures	
	Upper Denture	Lower Denture
Yawning:	%	%
Difficulties . .	4	7
None . . .	96	93
Talking:		
Difficulties . .	5	8
None . . .	95	92
Chewing meat:		
Difficulties . .	8	13
None . . .	92	87
Biting into a raw apple:		
Difficulties . .	21	25
None . . .	79	75
Fit of dentures:		
Too loose . .	16	25
About right .	83	74
Too tight . .	1	1
Comfort of dentures:		
Hurt . . .	4	12
Not . . .	96	88

Overall, lower dentures create more problems than upper dentures. The only sizeable problem for both plates appears to be biting into a raw apple.

Biting into a raw apple was by far the most difficult task for the fully-dentured, problems being encountered for 21% of upper dentures worn all day and 25% of lower dentures worn all day.

Very few dentures were thought to be too tight but considerable numbers were said to be too loose, and again it was the full lower denture which was the less satisfactory. Of those dentures worn all day the proportions which were too loose were 16% and 25% for upper and lower respectively.

There were however still some cases of the dentures being worn all day despite the problems they caused. Very few of the upper dentures that were worn were said to have made the person's mouth sore (4%), but 12% of lower dentures were said to have been troublesome in this respect.

The proportion of people with full dentures who wore them all the daytime and experienced none of the listed problems discussed was investigated. Of all those who had been fitted with full dentures just under a half (47%) wore them all day and had no problems. We asked the other 53% whether or not they were planning to visit the dentist to see if anything could be done about their dentures. 29% said they were planning to visit the dentist, and 71% said they were not. It would appear therefore that for many denture wearers the problems either did not seem particularly serious or they were fairly resigned to the situation continuing as it was.

8.4 The Circumstances of Total Tooth Loss

Since the event of full clearance is so final, and constitutes a mark of failure if the aim of the dental services is to enable adults to rely on natural teeth throughout most of life, the survey sought more details about the circumstances which surrounded the final loss of natural teeth. During the interview questions were asked concerning the situation at the time of, and prior to, the final extractions. This information is of course subject to memory, but all the evidence suggests that the occasion is a sufficient landmark in people's lives to be fairly reliably reported.

Among those who went to full dentures with no previous denture experience over a third lost more than twenty teeth, while another third lost fewer than twelve teeth. Even among those who did previously have a denture one in 10 said they lost more than twenty teeth at full clearance.

TABLE 8.12
The Number of Teeth Extracted at Full Clearance

Number of extracted	No previous denture experience	Previous denture experience	All
	%	%	%
1–11 . . .	34	59	41
12–20 . . .	31	31	31
21 or more . .	35	10	28
	100	100	100
BASES . .	265	99	364*

*Full denture wearers only, (5 people could not remember).

TABLE 8.13

The Number of Teeth Extracted at Full Clearance, by Age at Full Clearance

Number of teeth extracted	Age at full clearance (years)		All
	Less than 30	30 or over	
	%	%	%
1–11 . . .	24	47	42
12–20 . . .	34	29	30
21 or more . .	42	24	28
	100	100	100
BASES . .	86	300	386*†

*All edentulous.
†7 people could not remember.

There was some difference between the sexes in the proportion who had lost more than twenty teeth on the last occasion (Table 8.14). More women lost fewer than twelve teeth (44% of women lost fewer than 12 teeth compared to 39% for men). This difference reflects the fact that proportionally more women who became edentulous already had a denture. (Of those who previously had a denture 72% were women compared to 28% men). Proportionately more males lost over 20 teeth at full clearance (34%) compared with females (24%). The most noteable feature is that 60% of the edentulous studied were females.

TABLE 8.14

The Number of Teeth Extracted at Full Clearance, by Sex

Number of teeth extracted	Males	Females	All
	%	%	%
1–11 . . .	39	44	42
12–20 . . .	27	32	30
21 or more . .	34	24	28
	100	100	100
BASES . .	155	233	388*

*5 could not remember.

When asking about the time during which the informant still had some natural teeth, we asked whether he or she went to the dentist for a regular check-up, an occasional check-up, or only when having trouble (Table 8.15). 85% said they had only gone when having trouble, 8% said they had gone for an occasional check-up and 7% said they had gone for a regular check-up. It is difficult to compare the three groups since there were so few regular/occasional attenders. Regular attenders actually tended to lose more teeth, at full clearance, 71% losing 12 or more compared to 50% occasional and 58% who only went when having trouble.

TABLE 8.15

The Number of Teeth Extracted at Full Clearance, by Previous Dental Attendance

Number of teeth extracted	Previous attendance			
	Regular check-up	Occasional check-up	Only when having trouble	All
	%	%	%	%
1–11	29	50	42	41
12–20	39	25	30	31
21 or more	32	25	28	28
	100	100	100	100
BASES	28	32	325	385*

*7 could not remember; 1 never went for check-up.

A low proportion, 25% of those who had become edentulous in the 5 years before the survey said that they had never had any of their natural teeth filled. The number of teeth extracted differed slightly according to whether or not the person had ever had restorative treatment. Only 20 full denture wearers had lost all their teeth within the last 5 years. Slightly more of those who did not have restorative treatment lost over 20 teeth. If the groups are collated into 1–11 and 12+ teeth the results are almost exactly the same.

TABLE 8.16

The Number of Teeth Extracted at Full Clearance, by Whether Ever Had Fillings

Number of teeth extracted	Had fillings	Did not	All
	%	%	%
1–11	43	41	42
12–20	35	27	30
20 or more . . .	22	32	28
	100	100	100
BASES	160 (41%)	226 (59%)	386* (100%)

Base numbers re-weighted.
*Missing observations are as a result of some people being too old to remember.

In the interview we also asked if the informant suggested to the dentist that the teeth should be taken out or whether it was the dentist who suggested it. More people said that the dentist had suggested full clearance (32% said they had suggested it, and 60% said that the dentist had suggested it).* The number of teeth extracted varied slightly according to who suggested the extractions (Table 8.17). Proportionately more of those who suggested clearance themselves lost a smaller number of teeth. Nevertheless it appears that the decision to extract large numbers of teeth did not come from the patients alone, nor from the dentists alone.

TABLE 8.17

The Number of Teeth Extracted at Full Clearance, by Who Suggested Extraction

Number of teeth extracted	Informant suggested	Dentist suggested	All
	%	%	%
1–11	54	36	41
12–20	26	33	31
20 or more . . .	20	31	28
	100	100	100
BASES . . .	121	232	353*

Base numbers re-weighted.
*The other 8% were made up of: doctor/hospital suggested; mutual agreement; dont know/can't remember.

Perhaps the most striking result of this section is the high proportion of people who had massive extractions (28% lost over 20 and 58% lost over 12) and the high proportion who went straight to full clearance without ever having had dentures before.

TABLE 8.18

Fully Dentured Adults with No Previous Denture Experience

	%
Straight to full clearance	55
Series of visits	45
	100
BASE	265

Of **all** edentulous people, (Base 393), irrespective of whether or not they had full dentures, 59% went straight to a full clearance.

It has been stated that the transition from natural teeth to dentures should be a gradual process, commencing with a partial denture and progressing gradually to full dentures. This ideal is clearly far from being met at the present time.

8.5 The Cleansing of Full Dentures

No dental examinations of the edentulous were made during the survey, although full dentures were examined where there were some natural teeth present. Informants were however asked about denture hygiene. 17% found it difficult to clean dentures and 83% found no difficulty. 65% cleaned their teeth once per day, 35% twice or more. 62% cleaned their dentures by soaking, 68% by brushing and 1% by some other method. A large proportion, 75%, soaked their dentures in dental powder cleansers or solutions. Of persons who brushed their dentures 6% brushed them with soap, toothpaste was used by 56% and 18% used water as the main cleansing agent.

8.6 Denture Adhesives and Measures to Reduce Soreness

Of the edentulous persons interviewed for the survey only 14 people used a denture adhesive, of those, 13 used it on their bottom plate.

Full denture wearers were asked if they used anything to prevent or ease soreness. 5% said that they had used something and 95% said that they had not. Of those few who had used something, 29% had used tablets or lozenges to ease the soreness.

8.7 History of Dentures Currently in Use

Edentulous persons were asked how long ago they had been provided with their dentures.

TABLE 8.19

Length of Time since Dentures Were Fitted

	Male	Female
	%	%
Less than 2 years	4	12
2 years less than 5 years . . .	15	15
5 years less than 10 years . . .	25	18
10 years less than 20 years . . .	27	28
20 years or more	29	27

The vast majority of denture wearers had obtained them through the Health Service (80%) but a small proportion had obtained one or other plate privately (11%). 9% had obtained their dentures prior to 1948 when the Health Service came into being. Those who had obtained dentures privately were asked why. The main reasons were:—

(1) Dentures obtained privately are better quality   42%

(2) Wanted dentures quickly   16%

(3) Not available under NHS   16%

8.8 The Appearance of the Dentures

Edentulous persons were asked what they thought about the appearance of the dentures. 76% said that they were very satisfied, 14% that they were fairly satisfied, 6% not very satisfied and 4% not at all satisfied. Persons who were less than very satisfied were asked what features of the appearance of their denture did not satisfy them. 15% said the colour, 8% the shape, 20% that they did not look like their own natural teeth, and 19% that it was not the appearance so much as that they were ill fitting or uncomfortable.

8.9 Dentists Advice on Wearing Full Dentures

Advice from the dentist can help the new wearer of dentures to overcome the initial strangeness of the prosthesis. Persons who had been rendered edentulous less than ten years previously were asked what advice they had been given by the dentist when they first had dentures fitted.

TABLE 8.20

Dentists Advice on Wearing Full Dentures

	MALE			FEMALE		
	Yes	No	Can't Remember	Yes	No	Can't Remember
	%	%	%	%	%	%
Advice on chewing	16	81	3	6	84	10
Advice on biting	16	84	0	16	74	10
Advice on length of time to get used to dentures	31	63	6	29	55	16
Advice on length of time dentures could be expected to last	0	91	9	7	90	3
Advice on cleaning dentures	13	81	6	13	74	13
Advice on wearing dentures at night . . .	25	66	9	19	65	16

Base number re-weighted.

8.10 Reactions to New Full Dentures

Very few people (only 17% of the edentulous) had lost the last of their teeth within the last 10 years and it was this small group who were asked about the advice which their dentist had given them. In all of the above 6 categories the majority were not given any advice. Most advice would appear to be given on the length of time it would take to get used to the dentures. The proportion of full denture wearers who were given a leaflet about wearing dentures was 6%. 84% were not given a leaflet and 10% could not remember. It should be stated however that of those asked, 72% did not particularly want any more advice.

The length of time taken to get used to full dentures varied from less than one week (22%) to 1–3 months (57%). The majority (52%) took between 1 and 12 weeks to get used to wearing a denture. Most persons (72%) found nothing unexpected about wearing a denture. In particular it was found that 23% of those who did find something unexpected were conscious of their mouths feeling full.

8.11 Eating with New Full Dentures

Edentulous persons can sometimes experience differences in their eating habits when they begin to eat with full dentures. 9% of the full denture wearers interviewed said that they enjoyed their food more than before they had dentures. 67% about the same and 24% less than before they had them. Only 9% said that they had to change the kind of food they ate and 91% did not.

8.12 The Edentulous and the Loss of Natural Teeth

Persons who had lost all their teeth were asked how they felt about the loss of teeth at the time. 33% were upset/embarrassed and 50% were glad/untroubled. 58% of the edentulous had expected to lose their teeth at the age at which they were extracted but 35% were surprised to have lost all their teeth at that age. The advice which the edentulous would give to those who might soon have to have their remaining teeth extracted varied from 16% who would advise retaining the natural teeth, 39% who would advise clearance of the remaining natural teeth and 12% who would advise that the person should persevere with false teeth—"keep them in once they have been fitted".

8.13 Full Denture Wearers Who Had Previously Worn Dentures

Overall 26% of full denture wearers had previously worn dentures as shown in Table 8.21.

TABLE 8.21

Denture Worn Previously by Wearers of Full Dentures

	MALE				FEMALE				TOTAL
	N	S	E	W	N	S	E	W	
	%	%	%	%	%	%	%	%	%
Upper denture	100	100	100	57	74	93	74	86	81
Lower denture	0	0	0	0	9	0	11	0	5
Full denture	0	0	0	43	17	7	15	14	14
Of those with upper dentures:									
Full upper denture . .	40	20	17	25	65	38	25	17	41
Partial upper denture . .	60	80	83	75	35	62	75	83	59
Of those with lower dentures									
Full lower denture . .	So few had lower dentures which were worn previously that an overall picture only is appropriate.								24
Partial lower denture . .									76

In general, it would appear that the previous denture which was most commonly worn was a partial upper.

As well as information on the type of denture previously worn, the edentulous gave information on the number of sets of dentures worn previously. A large proportion, 87%, had worn one set only. Those who had worn more than one set were asked about the other sets. 94% had a top plate only, none had worn a lower only and 6% had both. Of those who had an upper plate or both, 39% had a full upper plate and 61% a partial.

8.14 Appearance Without Full Dentures

Some people are sensitive to being seen without their full dentures. Of those wearing their dentures at the time of interview 22% stated that they were very much worried by their family seeing them without teeth. 20% to some extent and 49% not at all. 5% had no family. (4% were not wearing their dentures at the time of interview).

So far as people outside the family seeing them without their teeth were concerned 45% were very much worried, 22% to some extent and 33% not at all.

8.15 Extraction of the Remaining Teeth

Reference has previously been made to the circumstances of total tooth loss.

There were regional variations in the number of teeth extracted at the final clearance as is shown in Table 8.22.

TABLE 8.22

Extraction of Remaining Teeth

	MALE				FEMALE			
	N	S	E	W	N	S	E	W
	%	%	%	%	%	%	%	%
Number of teeth extracted:								
1–11	41	50	27	54	48	53	29	41
12–20	26	36	29	14	46	35	25	38
21 or more	33	14	44	32	6	12	36	21

60% of persons had their remaining teeth extracted all in one visit and 40% during a series of visits.

72% had their teeth extracted because their teeth were decayed, 26% because the gums were bad and 2% for some other reason such as:

(1) Teeth were loose/falling out/coming away from the gums

(2) Asked to have them out even though they could have been saved } Only 0.5% each

(3) Teeth were affecting general health

24% who had all their remaining teeth removed found the experience very upsetting, 25% a little upsetting and 51% not at all upsetting.

8.16 Replacement of the Remaining Teeth

16% of full denture wearers had a denture fitted the same day as they had their remaining teeth extracted, 24% up to one month later, 29% between one month and three months afterwards, 21% between three and six months and 10% more than six months later.

9. Choice and Continuity in the Dental Services

9.1 Choice of Dentist

The reason why persons choose a particular dentist is of interest. It can have a bearing upon the provision of dental facilities for a health centre for example. The survey investigated the reasons why persons chose to attend a particular dentist. The results are summarised in Table 9.1.

TABLE 9.1

Reasons for Choosing a Particular Dentist

	Northern	Southern	Eastern	Western	All
	%	%	%	%	%
Nearest	31	13	23	17	22
Recommended by relative/friend . . .	30	22	32	35	30
Family dentist	18	30	20	23	22
Only one/first one found	4	6	2	10	5
Recommended by doctor/another dentist .	4	3	3	1	3
Just by chance	3	3	1	1	2
Works dentist/hospital	1	2	0	1	1
Letter	7	18	18	9	13
Specialist	2	3	1	3	2
TOTAL	100	100	100	100	100

Base: 964.

9.2 Continuity

The continuity of the attachment to a particular dentist is also of interest. General dental practitioners, unlike medical practitioners in the Health Service, accept patients for a course of treatment only. They do not have a list of patients in the same way that their medical colleagues do. Despite this, many persons regard themselves as the patient of a particular general dental practitioner and consult that practitioner about their dental health, sometimes over many years. Of the persons interviewed, 70% had been to the same dentist or group of dentists previously. The group which was returning to the same dental practice was asked to provide further information relevant to regular attendance. Two per cent had been attending that particular dentist for less than a year, 28% one year but less than 5 and 65% 5 years or more. Five per cent did not know or could not remember.

9.3 Reminders

Some dentists remind patients to return for a dental examination usually 6 months after a course of treatment. Informants were asked to provide information about reminders. Thirty-five per cent stated that the dentist sends a reminder. Persons who did not receive a reminder or who had attended the dentist for the first time were asked how they arranged their next examination. Ten per cent arranged an appointment at the end of a previous course of treatment, 35% sometime before the date of the appointment and 54% when they wanted to see the dentist as soon as possible. Other reasons were given also.

9.4 Waiting for Appointments

The time which persons seeking dental treatment had to wait showed a variation as shown in Table 9.2.

TABLE 9.2

Length of Time Waiting for a Dental Appointment

	Northern	Southern	Eastern	Western	All
	%	%	%	%	%
Same day	18	27	18	25	21
Less than one week	23	11	25	18	20
One week, less than two	15	21	19	20	19
Two weeks, less than three	11	9	10	8	10
Three weeks, less than four	4	5	4	3	4
One month	8	7	4	6	6
More than one month	4	12	3	9	6
Different appointment arranged . . .	0	1	1	2	1
Don't know	17	7	16	9	12

10. Private Treatment

The Department of Health and Social Services is responsible for the Health Services in Northern Ireland. Its responsibility includes dental care in the hospital, community and general dental services. It does not include dental treatment provided under a private arrangement between patient and dental practitioner. Because of the possible effects which a growth in private treatment could have upon the general dental services the Department is interested in the extent to which private treatment is being provided. As the normal monitoring processes do not apply to private treatment, the survey was considered to provide an opportunity of providing information.

There has been reason to believe that dental treatment under private contract has increased in recent years.

Informants who were non-dentate as well as informants who were dentate were asked to provide information about private dental care. The information gave some indication of the extent of private dental treatment in Northern Ireland. The results are presented in relation to sex and social class (Table 10.1). It would appear that private dental treatment is a small component of dental care in Northern Ireland. Only 75 people of the total sample of 1,176 had had private dental treatment. (Table 10.4).

TABLE 10.1

Persons who have had All or Some Private Dental Treatment

| | Household Social Class | | | | | | | |
| | I, II and III Non-manual | | III Manual | | IV Non-manual, IV Manual and V | | All Social Classes | |
	M	F	M	F	M	F	M	F
	%	%	%	%	%	%	%	%
Wanted treatment done privately . . .	61	50	0		50	39	58	42
Would have preferred Health Service dentistry .	39	50	0		50	61	42	58
Asked the dentist if he would do Health Service dentistry	45	50	0		67	67	44	36
Did not ask the dentist if he would do Health Service dentistry	55	50	0		33	33	56	64
Given reasons for not being able to obtain Health Service treatment	57	33	0		33	80	33	62
Not given reasons for not being able to obtain Health Service treatment . . .	43	67	0		67	20	67	38

Bases vary for each question as few persons had private treatment.

Not all the dental treatment which is provided outside the general dental services is private treatment. Table 10.2 shows the percentages of treatment outside the general dental services.

The type of treatment provided privately was also of interest. For this reason Table 10.3 gives the various types of private treatment provided.

Reasons for having dental treatment privately rather than under the Health Service can exist. Informants were asked for their reasons for obtaining private dental treatment. These reasons are shown in Table 10.4.

TABLE 10.2

General Dental Service Dental Treatment and Other Methods of Providing Treatment

All Adults	%
Health Service (GDS)	90
Private	8
Health Service plus private	1
Community dental service	
Armed services . . . . . . }	1
Other	
TOTAL	100
BASE	973*

*The dentate plus those edentulous who had visited a dentist within the last ten years.

TABLE 10.3

Type of Treatment Provided Privately for All Adults

	%
Bridgework	} 20
Crowns	
Dentures	10
Extractions	30
Fillings	30
Intravenous Anaesthetic	10
Other	—

TABLE 10.4

The Reason for Obtaining Private Dental Treatment

All Adults who had Private Treatment	%
1. Wanted better quality treatment	25
2. Treatment not available under Health Service	17
3. Wanted treatment quickly	24
4. Dentist does not provide treatment under the Health Service	17
5. Other	17
TOTAL	100
BASE	75*

*Very few people actually had private treatment.

11. Public Attitudes to the Type and Availability of Dental Services

11.1 Difficulty in Obtaining Dental Services

The survey examined the ease or difficulty of obtaining dental services. In general it would seem that dental treatment is fairly easy to obtain. In order to provide local information, the results were calculated on the basis of the Health and Social Services Board Areas, Northern, Southern, Eastern and Western (Table 11.1).

TABLE 11.1

Attitudes to the Availability of Health Service Dental Treatment

	Northern	Southern	Eastern	Western	All
	%	%	%	%	%
Very easy to obtain treatment . . .	41	29	52	39	43
Fairly easy	34	37	29	37	32
Fairly difficult	4	10	2	6	5
Very difficult	5	10	2	5	5
Don't know/No opinion . . .	16	14	15	13	15
TOTAL	100	100	100	100	100
BASE	268	233	501	174	1,176

11.2 Distance from Dental Services

The survey sought information on the distance, type of transport and length of time necessary to visit the dentist. Table 11.2 summarises the results. 47% of the informants considered the dental surgery very convenient and 2% very inconvenient. Most people (87%) considered it very convenient or fairly convenient.

TABLE 11.2

Distance, Transport and Time from Residence to Dental Surgery

	Northern	Southern	Eastern	Western	All
	%	%	%	%	%
Less than 1 mile	25	20	32	23	27
1 mile less than 2	20	21	32	14	24
2 miles less than 5	27	17	17	21	20
5 miles less than 10	20	32	5	18	16
More than 10	5	9	5	23	8
Don't know	3	1	9	1	5
	100	100	100	100	100
	%	%	%	%	%
Walk	26	23	41	22	31
Public Transport	14	17	13	17	15
Car/Motor cycle	46	44	35	38	40
Driven by another	12	16	8	21	12
Bicycle	1	0	0	1	0
Other	1	0	3	1	2
	100	100	100	100	100
	%	%	%	%	%
Approx. 5 minutes	16	10	24	12	17
Approx. 10 minutes	30	30	30	20	29
Approx. 15 minutes	28	21	18	17	21
Approx. 20 minutes	10	22	9	24	14
More than 20 minutes	14	15	10	26	14
Don't know	2	2	9	1	5
	100	100	100	100	100
BASES	268	233	501	174	1,176

11.3 The Availability of Emergency Dental Treatment

A body which has the responsibility of providing dental services is conscious of the need which may arise for emergency dental services. Sudden severe toothache, trauma and haemorrhage can cause persons to seek dental treatment outside normal surgery hours.

4% of persons had sought emergency dental treatment during the last 5 years. Of this number 56% had sought the treatment within the last 2 years. Most people (95%) sought treatment within 3 days, mostly (51%) on a week day, 26% on a Saturday and 23% on a Sunday or a Bank Holiday. The most common time to seek treatment (48%) was between 9 o'clock and 12 o'clock, although a fairly large number (25%) sought treatment between 12 o'clock and 6 o'clock. Most people (92%) sought treatment from an ordinary dental surgeon, and had been to that dentist previously.

A significant proportion of persons (30%) did not succeed in obtaining dental treatment the same day. 10% obtained treatment the next day, 10% 2–3 days later and 10% 4 or more days later. Most people were satisfied (83%) but some 17% were dissatisfied with the time which they had to wait.

Further information was sought from persons who were unable to obtain emergency dental treatment from the dentist whom they first approached. 60% did something else and 40% just waited. Most people (57%) obtained treatment the same day. The percentages were 57% treated the same day, 9% the next day, 24% waited 2–3 days and 5% had to wait more than 3 days. 5% did not know or could not remember.

A fairly high degree of satisfaction was expressed at the promptness of treatment. 44% were very satisfied, 17% fairly satisfied, 11% fairly dissatisfied and 28% very dissatisfied.

11.4 Attitudes to Dental Services for Children

Parents of children may have to decide between obtaining treatment for their children from general dental practitioners or from dental officers of the community dental services. The Department provides funds for these services and thus information on public attitudes to the services is of interest to the Department.

General dental practitioners are independent dentists who enter into a contract with one of the Health and Social Services Boards to provide dental treatment under the General Dental Services Regulations. They provide most Health Service dental treatment. They provide their own premises, equipment and staff. The standard of dental treatment is monitored on behalf of the Boards by the Central Services Agency.

The community dental services provide the school dental service. Dental officers visit schools to provide school inspections. Children requiring dental care can be offered treatment, either at a dental clinic or in a mobile dental clinic brought to the school. The community dental services are provided by the Health and Social Services Boards who employ staff and provide facilities. The service does not however extend to all schools. Due to insufficient numbers of dental staff only a proportion of schools is served by the dental service.

Although the survey was concerned with adult dental health, the attitudes of the adult population can be expected to influence the dental health of children. For that reason adults were asked questions about dental services for children.

19% said that they would prefer children to receive dental treatment by means of a mobile dental caravan visiting the school, 18% by children visiting a dental clinic and 45% by children visiting a health service dentist at his own surgery. 18% did not know or had no opinion.

11.5 Attitudes to the Different Branches of the Dental Services

Although most members of the public are accustomed to obtaining dental treatment through general dental services an increasing number is coming into contact with other branches of the dental services. The hospital dental service has expanded in recent years and the community dental service can now treat the adult handicapped.

Informants were questioned about their attitudes to the different branches of the dental services, and whether they considered them satisfactory. Most people (78%) considered that the general dental service was satisfactory. Some (11%) considered it unsatisfactory but 11% did not know or had no opinion. 43% considered school services as satisfactory, 7% unsatisfactory while 50% did not know. Services for the handicapped were considered satisfactory by 12%, unsatisfactory by 1% while most (87%) did not know or had no opinion.

12. Preferences for Dental Treatment

12.1 Preferences for the Treatment of Natural Teeth

We asked all those people who still had some natural teeth whether, if they had an aching tooth, they would prefer the tooth to be extracted or filled. This was asked separately for back teeth and front teeth. The overall preferences for the two kinds of treatment are given in Table 12.1.

TABLE 12.1

Preference for Extractions versus Fillings for Adults With Some Natural Teeth

Preference for extractions versus fillings if a tooth was aching	Adults with some natural teeth	
	Back tooth	Front tooth
	%	%
Have it out	38	15
Have it filled	60	84
Other answer	2	1
	100	100
BASE	783	

Base number re-weighted.

For the aching back tooth, while 60% of people said that they would prefer it to be filled, 38% said they would prefer it to be extracted. A small proportion of people (2%) gave some other qualified answer, for example, that it would depend on the state of the tooth or that they would let the dentist decide. Thus conservation of an aching back tooth did not seem important for many people. For the aching front tooth the situation was different, and appearance seemed to play an important part; almost all (84%) said that they would prefer the tooth to be filled. Nevertheless (15%) said they would prefer extraction. As with the aching back tooth 1% of people gave some other qualified answer.

In previous chapters it was found that dental attitudes and dental health vary for different groups of people, and next investigated was how the preferences for extractions versus fillings vary for people of different ages, sexes, social classes and dental attendance patterns.

TABLE 12.2

Preference for Extractions versus Fillings, for Adults of Different Ages

Preference for extractions versus fillings if a back tooth was aching	Adults with some natural teeth					
	Present age					
	16–24	25–34	35–44	45–54	55 and over	All ages
	%	%	%	%	%	%
Have it out	39	33	35	31	55	38
Have it filled	59	65	63	68	42	60
Other answer	2	2	2	1	3	2
	100	100	100	100	100	100
Preference for extractions versus fillings if a front tooth was aching	%	%	%	%	%	%
Have it out	8	11	8	16	37	15
Have it filled	91	88	91	82	59	84
Other answer	1	1	1	2	4	1
	100	100	100	100	100	100
BASES	182	186	162	121	132	783

Base numbers re-weighted.

Below 55 years, age did not seem to have much bearing on whether a person preferred an aching tooth to be extracted (Table 12.2), and this was so both for the aching back tooth and the aching front tooth. It is unfortunate that attitudes towards conservative dental treatment at the present time are such that even among the youngest adults (16–24) 39% said they would prefer an aching back tooth to be extracted and 8% said that they would prefer an aching front tooth to be extracted.

It has been seen earlier that more women in the most dentate age groups (Table 5.23) go to the dentist for a regular check-up and that women have more evidence of restorative treatment than men. It might therefore be expected that preferences for treatment would differ for men and women, but Table 12.3 shows that it is only in terms of an aching front tooth that the sexes differed significantly. Almost one fifth (19%) of men said they would prefer an aching front tooth to be extracted compared to 11% of women. Appearance would appear to play a more important part for the women.

Table 12.4 gives the preferences for extractions versus fillings for the three main social class groups, and the differences between the different social classes were substantial. In the top social class group, (I, II and III non-manual) comparatively few people said they would prefer extraction of the aching tooth, even an aching back tooth; the proportions preferring extraction were 23% and 10% for back and front respectively. This contrasts with people in the lowest social class group (IV and V), among whom 51% said they would prefer extraction of the aching back tooth and 21% said they would prefer extraction of the aching front tooth. People in the intermediate social class group (III manual) were somewhat more like people in the lowest social class group in terms of their preferences.

TABLE 12.3

Preference for Extractions versus Fillings for Different Sexes

Preference for extractions versus fillings if a back tooth was aching	Adults with some natural teeth		
	Male	Female	All
	%	%	%
Have it out	40	36	38
Have it filled	57	62	60
Other answer	3	2	2
	100	100	100
Preference for extractions versus fillings if a front tooth was aching	%	%	%
Have it out	19	11	15
Have it filled	79	88	83
Other answer	2	1	2
	100	100	100
BASES	378	405	783

Base numbers re-weighted.

TABLE 12.4

Preference for Extractions versus Fillings, for Different Social Classes

Preference for extractions versus fillings if a back tooth was aching	Adults with some natural teeth				
	Household social class				
	I, II and III non-manual	III manual	IV non-manual, IV manual and V	Housewife	All* social classes
	%	%	%	%	%
Have it out	23	44	51	42	38
Have it filled	75	55	47	57	60
Other answer	2	1	2	1	2
	100	100	100	100	100
Preference for extractions versus fillings if a front tooth was aching	%	%	%	%	%
Have it out	10	17	21	12	15
Have it filled	88	83	77	87	84
Other answer	2	0	2	1	1
	100	100	100	100	100
BASES	250	185	131	145	783

Base numbers re-weighted.

*Includes the student, unemployed and unclassifiable categories which are not included elsewhere in the table.

As we would expect, the preferences for adults with different dental attendance patterns were quite different (Table 12.5). Among those who attended for a regular check-up only 15% said they would prefer an aching back tooth to be extracted, and only 3% said they would prefer an aching front tooth to be extracted. Thus the preference for restorative treatment of the front tooth was almost universal among the regular attenders, 95% saying they would prefer the aching front tooth to be filled. The situation for the irregular attenders was quite different, 59% saying they would prefer the aching back tooth to be taken out and 27% saying they would prefer an aching front tooth to be taken out.

TABLE 12.5

Preference for Extractions versus Fillings, for Different Attendance Patterns

	Adults with some natural teeth			
Preference for extractions versus fillings if a back tooth was aching	Regular check-up	Occasional check-up	Only when have trouble	All
	%	%	%	%
Have it out	15	22	59	38
Have it filled	81	78	40	60
Other answer	4	0	1	2
	100	100	100	100
Preference for extractions versus fillings if a front tooth was aching	%	%	%	%
Have it out	3	3	27	15
Have it filled	95	97	71	83
Other answer	2	0	2	2
	100	100	100	100
BASES	298	98	387	783

Base numbers re-weighted.

Having already seen that social class and dental attendance pattern are both important in terms of whether extractions or fillings are preferred for aching teeth, it is of value to look at the situation for different social classes and attendance patterns to see if they are acting independently and, if so, which seems to be the more important. If they are indeed acting independently then one would expect the least preference for extractions (and conversely the greatest preference for fillings) among the regular attenders of the top social class groups and the greatest preference for extractions of aching teeth among the irregular attenders of the lowest social class groups. This is in fact the case, as is shown in Table 12.6 (so that the table should be manageable, the preferences are summarised in terms of the proportion who would prefer extraction).

For an aching back tooth the proportion who said they would prefer the tooth to be extracted ranged from 13% among the regular attenders of the top social class groups to 79% among the irregular attenders of the lowest social class groups. Attendance pattern had a somewhat greater effect than social class, the range for the different attendance patterns being 19% to 29% to 72%, and the range for the different social classes being 23% to 44% to 51%.

Similarly there was a large difference in the proportion who said they would prefer an aching front tooth to be extracted. Only 2% of the regular attenders of the top social class groups said they would prefer extraction, compared to 37% of the irregular attenders of the manual groups. Again dental attendance seemed to have somewhat more effect than social class, in that only 3% of people with the most favourable attendance pattern (ie the regular attenders) said they would prefer extraction for the aching front tooth compared to 37% of irregular attenders, the range for different social classes being 10% to 17% to 21%.

TABLE 12.6

Preference for Extractions versus Fillings, by Attendance Pattern and Social Class

Aching back tooth	Adults with some natural teeth			
	Proportion would would prefer an aching tooth to be extracted*			
	Regular check-up	Occasional check-up	Only when have trouble	Overall rates for social classes
	%	%	%	%
S.C. I, II, III non-manual . . .	13	13	59	23	
S.C. III manual	20	35	85	44	from
S.C. IV and V	35	53	79	51	Table
Housewife	21	29	82	42	12.4
Other	26	—	49	42	
Overall rates by attendance pattern from Table 12.5	15	22	59	38
Aching front tooth				
S.C. I, II, III non-manual . .	2	—	31	10	
S.C. III manual	9	—	37	17	from
S.C. IV and V	5	13	37	21	Table
Housewife	2	7	29	12	12.4
Other	—	—	29	20	
Overall rates by attendance pattern from Table 12.5	3	3	27	15

Base numbers re-weighted.

*Calculated as follows:—

$$\frac{\text{Number of people in the group preferring extraction}}{\text{Number of people in each cell}} \times 100 = \text{Rate} — \text{for example:—}$$

$$\frac{\text{Total number of regular attenders who said that they preferred extraction}}{\text{Total number of regular attenders}}$$

Although there were some regular attenders who said they would prefer an extraction, and conversely some irregular attenders who said they would prefer a filling (especially in the case of an aching front tooth), it is obvious that the overall preferences of the regular dental attenders are destined to preserve them as being dentate adults, while the preferences of the irregular attenders can do nothing but hasten the event of total tooth loss.

It is difficult to assess the extent to which these preferences would actually affect the decision for the treatment of an aching tooth, or even whether having an aching tooth is a situation with which the person was familiar. It can be expected however, that the stated preferences would have some bearing on the dental treatment which the person was in the habit of receiving. This was investigated in two ways, firstly by examining the dental condition of the mouth. This showed the result of all past dental disease and treatment. Secondly the interview investigated the treatment which the person claimed to have received when he or she last visited the dentist.

The preference for extraction versus restorative treatment and the dental condition itself varied according to dental attendance pattern. The relationship between the dental condition and the preferred treatment, whether the person goes to the dentist for a regular check-up or only when in trouble was investigated. Since the preferences vary in a similar way, for back teeth or for front teeth, the analysis is confined to the dental condition according to back tooth preference.

Table 12.7 gives the numbers of missing teeth according to dental attendance pattern and the preference for the treatment of an aching back tooth. People who said they would prefer the tooth to be extracted had more missing teeth than those who said they would prefer restorative treatment, this being equally so for the regular and the irregular attenders. For example, the regular attenders who said they would prefer an extraction had, on average, 8.7 missing teeth, and almost a quarter (24%) of them had 12 or more missing teeth. The corresponding figures for the regular attenders who said they would prefer the tooth to be filled were 8.2 and 20% respectively. Among the irregular attenders the overall tooth loss was, of course, greater than among the regular attenders, but those irregular attenders who said they would prefer extraction were in a worse position than those who said they would prefer restorative treatment; for example those preferring extraction had 13.4 missing teeth on average, and 14% had 5 or fewer missing teeth, the figures for those preferring fillings being 8.9 and 31% respectively.

TABLE 12.7

The Number of Missing Teeth, by Dental Attendance and Preference for Back Tooth Treatment

Number of missing teeth	Adults with some natural teeth			
	Regular check-up		Only when having trouble	
	Have aching back tooth out	Have aching back tooth filled	Have aching back tooth out	Have aching back tooth filled
	%	%	%	%
0	0	3	1	2
1– 5	41	34	13	29
6–11	35	43	34	42
12–17	16	10	23	17
18 or more	8	10	29	10
	100	100	100	100
Average number of missing teeth .	8.7	8.2	13.4	8.9
BASES	37	182	178	167

Base numbers re-weighted.

Table 12.8 shows that 3% of the regular attenders who said they would prefer an aching back tooth to be extracted had no filled teeth, compared to 1% of the regular attenders who said they would prefer the tooth to be filled. The average numbers of filled teeth were 9.6 and 12.0 respectively. Among the irregular attenders (who had less evidence of restorative treatment than the regular attenders) 32% of those who said they would prefer extraction of the aching back tooth had no filled teeth, compared to only 10% of the irregular attenders who said they would prefer restorative treatment. The average numbers of filled teeth for these two groups of irregular attenders were 4.5 and 8.3 respectively.

TABLE 12.8

The Number of Filled, Otherwise Sound Teeth, by Dental Attendance and Preference for Back Tooth Treatment

Number of filled teeth	Adults with some natural teeth			
	Regular check-up		Only when having trouble	
	Have aching back tooth out	Have aching back tooth filled	Have aching back tooth out	Have aching back tooth filled
	%	%	%	%
0	3	1	32	10
1– 5	13	8	31	22
6–11	46	39	26	40
12–17	30	38	11	23
18 or more	8	14	0	5
	100	100	100	100
Average number of filled teeth .	9.6	12.0	4.5	8.3
BASES	37	182	178	167

Base numbers re-weighted.

It is difficult to tell how much of the relationships which we have found in Tables 12.7 and 12.8 are direct ones, because in many cases teeth will not be aching when the person goes to the dentist. But similar attitudes may well exist towards teeth which have less severe decay, and it is these attitudes which play a contributory role each time the person visits the dentist. In this respect it is of interest to look at the treatment the person received in the last course of treatment, and the results are given in Table 12.9.

TABLE 12.9

Major Type of Treatment Received at Last Visit, by Preference for Back Tooth Treatment

Treatment received in the last course of treatment	Adults with some natural teeth	
	Have aching back tooth filled	Have aching back tooth out
	%	%
Toothache	79	88
Fillings	11	4
Loose teeth	3	1
Broken teeth	6	6
Other	1	1
	100	100
BASES	188	223

Base numbers re-weighted.

The bases drop because not all people had had dental treatment and so were not asked what it was.

12.2   Attitudes Towards Having Dentures

In this section preferences for dental treatment and peoples' attitudes towards having dentures are investigated. All adults who still relied wholly on natural teeth were asked whether, if they were to lose some of their own teeth and needed dentures to replace them, they would find the thought of having partial dentures very upsetting, a little upsetting or not at all upsetting (Table 12.10).

TABLE 12.10

Attitudes to Having Partial Dentures in Conjunction with Natural Teeth, by Dental Attendance Pattern

Finds the thought of having a partial denture	Adults who rely wholly on natural teeth			
	Regular check-up	Occasional check-up	Only when have trouble	All
	%	%	%	%
Very upsetting	38	40	25	33
A little upsetting	35	22	26	29
Not at all upsetting . . .	27	38	49	38
	100	100	100	100
BASES	223	80	247	550*

Base numbers re-weighted.

*Only asked of people who relied wholly on natural teeth.

Dentate adults were fairly evenly split according to how they viewed the thought of eventually having full dentures: (Table 12.11), 54% said they found the thought very upsetting, 22% said they found it a little upsetting and 24% said they found the thought not at all upsetting. As we might expect, there were considerable differences according to dental attendance pattern, and it was the irregular attenders who had markedly different views on the subject. Thirty-four per cent of those dentate adults who went to the dentist only when they were having trouble said they found the thought of having full dentures not at all upsetting, compared to 12% of the regular attenders. Conversely 44% of the irregular attenders found the thought very upsetting compared to 65% of the regular attenders. Thus despite the more ready acceptance of full dentures among those with the least favourable dental attendance pattern, even among the regular attenders some did not find the thought of full dentures at all upsetting.

We looked at how people found the thought of having full dentures, for different age groups. More of the youngest adults found the thought very upsetting (60%) compared to the oldest adults. Thirty-three per cent of those aged 55 and over found the thought of full dentures very upsetting. Conversely the proportions who found the thought not at all upsetting were 21% and 43% respectively. Those dentate adults who had no previous denture experience tended to find the thought of having full dentures somewhat more upsetting than those who already had been provided with dentures to complement their natural teeth: 60% of those wholly reliant on natural teeth found the thought of full dentures very upsetting compared with 40% of the partially-dentured. Conversely the proportions finding the thought of full dentures not at all upsetting were 21% and 31% respectively.

TABLE 12.11
Attitudes to Full Dentures, by Dental Attendance Pattern

Finds the thought of having full dentures:	Adults with some natural teeth			
	Regular check-up	Occasional check-up	Only when have trouble	All
	%	%	%	%
Very upsetting	65	63	44	54
A little upsetting	23	18	22	22
Not at all upsetting	12	19	34	24
	100	100	100	100
BASES	298	98	387	783

Base numbers re-weighted.

The large numbers of people who would prefer the extraction of an aching tooth, or who accept total tooth loss and full dentures, indicate the low priority given to reliance on natural teeth. The improvement of public attitudes to the retention of the natural dentition will require more than the mere encouragement of people to go to the dentist regularly. We have seen in this chapter that even among the regular attenders there are people whose preferences for treatment and attitudes on dentures do not favour the retention of the natural teeth.

13. Cleaning Natural Teeth

During the interview all people who still had some natural teeth were asked a series of questions about cleaning them and in this chapter the frequency and methods of cleaning and whether a dentist had ever demonstrated to them how best to clean their teeth are examined.

13.1 The Frequency of Tooth Cleaning, by Attendance Pattern, Age, Sex and Social Class

People varied greatly in the frequency with which they said they cleaned their natural teeth. There was a small proportion (2%) whose interest in their oral hygiene was obviously very low, since they said they never cleaned their natural teeth at all; 9% said they cleaned their teeth less than once a day, 32% said they cleaned them once a day, 42% said they cleaned them twice a day and 13% said they cleaned them three or more times a day.* The variation in frequency of cleaning for the different dental attendance patterns was quite considerable (Table 13.1). Among the regular dental attenders only 2% cleaned their teeth less than once a day, and just about one fifth (19%) said they cleaned them three or more times a day. The irregular attenders who attended only when they were having trouble showed much less frequent tooth cleaning. 4% said they never cleaned their teeth, 13% said they cleaned them less than once a day, and only 9% said they cleaned them three or more times a day. The occasional attenders cleaned their teeth more often than the irregular attenders but not as often as those who went to the dentist for a regular check-up.

TABLE 13.1

Frequency of Tooth Cleaning, by Dental Attendance Pattern

Frequency of cleaning natural teeth	Adults with some natural teeth			
	Regular check-up	Occasional check-up	Only when having trouble	All
	%	%	%	%
Never	—	—	4	2
Less than daily	2	3	13	9
Once daily	24	32	39	32
Twice daily	55	49	30	42
Three or more times daily	19	16	9	13
Other	—	—	5	2
	100	100	100	100
BASES	298	98	387	783

Base numbers re-weighted.

Men and women had somewhat different frequencies of tooth cleaning, men cleaning their teeth less often on average than women. Among men who still had some natural teeth 3% said they never cleaned their teeth and 14% said they cleaned them less than once a day, these proportions for women being 1% and 2% respectively. The proportions who cleaned their teeth three or more times a day were 8% and 18% for men and women respectively.

*2% gave other answers.

72

Table 13.2 gives the results for different attendance patterns and sexes. As we would expect, the female regular attender had the highest frequency of tooth cleaning and male irregular attenders the lowest. Just under a quarter (20%) of the women who attended the dentist for a regular check-up said they cleaned their teeth three or more times a day, compared to only 4% of men who attended only when they had trouble. Conversely only 1% of the female regular attenders cleaned their teeth less than daily, whereas among the men who attended only when they had trouble, (19%) cleaned their teeth less than daily and 5% said they never cleaned them.

TABLE 13.2

Frequency of Tooth Cleaning, by Dental Attendance Pattern and Sex

Frequency of cleaning natural teeth	Adults with some natural teeth							
	Regular check-up		Occasional check-up		Only when having trouble		All	
	M	F	M	F	M	F	M	F
	%	%	%	%	%	%	%	%
Never	—	—	—	—	5	2	3	1
Less than daily	3	1	9	—	19	4	14	2
Once daily	30	21	46	24	41	37	38	27
Twice daily	50	58	34	58	25	38	33	50
Three or more times daily . .	17	20	11	18	4	16	8	18
Other	—	—	—	—	6	3	4	2
	100	100	100	100	100	100	100	100
BASES	115	183	36	62	226	161	377	406

Base number re-weighted.

The frequency of tooth cleaning for the different social classes was investigated. People in the top social class group cleaned their teeth more often than people in the other two social class groups (Table 13.3). There was little difference between the intermediate social class group (III manual) and the lowest social class group (IV and V) in the overall pattern of tooth cleaning. Only 5% of people in the top social class group cleaned their natural teeth less than daily compared to 12% and 11% in the other two social class groups; conversely the proportions who cleaned their teeth three or more times a day were 18%, 9% and 10% respectively.

The frequency of teeth cleaning for people of different ages was also investigated and (Table 13.4) the only difference was that more people in the oldest age group (55 and over) said they never cleaned their teeth (7% compared to 1% among those aged 16–34 and 0% among those aged 35–44).

TABLE 13.3

Frequency of Tooth Cleaning, by Household Social Class

Frequency of cleaning natural teeth	Adults with some natural teeth				
	Household social class				
	I, II and non-manual	III manual	IV non-manual, IV manual and V	Housewife	All* social classes
	%	%	%	%	%
Never	1	2	4	1	2
Once a day . . .	28	37	31	34	33
Twice a day . . .	47	37	39	48	42
More than twice daily .	18	9	10	13	13
Less than once daily . .	5	12	11	2	8
Other	1	3	5	2	2
	100	100	100	100	100
BASES	257	185	132	145	783

Base numbers re-weighted.

*Includes the student, unemployed and unclassifiable categories which are not included elsewhere in the table.

TABLE 13.4
Frequency of Tooth Cleaning by Age

Frequency of cleaning natural teeth	Adults with some natural teeth					
	16–24	25–34	35–44	45–54	55+	All ages
	%	%	%	%	%	%
Never	1	1	—	2	7	2
Less than daily	6	8	9	5	10	8
Once daily	33	36	33	26	32	33
Twice daily	44	42	43	49	32	42
More than twice daily . . .	14	12	14	16	11	13
Other	2	1	1	2	8	2
TOTAL	100	100	100	100	100	100
BASE	182	186	162	121	132	783

13.2 Methods of Tooth Cleaning

The survey investigated the timing of the first two occasions of tooth cleaning in order to examine the possibility of a correlation between tooth cleaning times and dental disease.

TABLE 13.5A

The Timing of Tooth Cleaning Among Dentate Adults (First Occasion)

Time of cleaning	Adults with some natural teeth											
	16–24		25–34		35–44		45–54		55+		All Ages	
	M	F	M	F	M	F	M	F	M	F	M	F
	%	%	%	%	%	%	%	%	%	%	%	%
Before breakfast . . .	33	26	30	32	45	24	40	40	39	28	36	29
After breakfast . . .	29	67	43	53	33	70	33	51	37	55	35	60
Mid-day	2	—	—	2	1	2	6	—	—	—	2	1
Tea time	5	—	1	1	—	—	—	—	—	—	1	—
After evening meal . .	9	1	1	1	6	—	6	—	2	—	5	1
Last thing at night . .	19	6	19	9	11	4	13	7	14	14	16	8
Other (inc. no particular time) .	3	—	6	2	4	—	2	2	8	3	5	1
	100		100		100		100		100		100	
BASE	88	93	86	98	75	87	59	59	59	64	367	401*

*Those who never cleaned their teeth were not asked about timing.

TABLE 13.5B

The Timing of Tooth Cleaning Among Dentate Adults (Second Occasion)

Time of cleaning	Adults with some natural teeth											
	16–24		25–34		35–44		45–54		55+		All ages	
	M	F	M	F	M	F	M	F	M	F	M	F
	%	%	%	%	%	%	%	%	%	%	%	%
Before breakfast . . .	—	—	—	—	—	—	—	—	—	—	—	—
After breakfast . . .	3	1	—	5	—	4	8	5	—	8	2	4
Mid-day	3	11	6	15	13	15	17	11	24	21	11	14
Tea time	12	6	3	4	7	7	4	5	—	4	6	5
After evening meal . .	20	16	20	10	7	15	25	11	—	4	16	13
Last thing at night . .	62	66	71	66	70	57	46	68	76	63	65	64
Other	—	—	—	—	3	2	—	—	—	—	—	—
	100		100		100		100		100		100	
BASE	34	70	35	59	30	53	24	37	17	24	140	243*

*Only 383 people actually gave a second occasion on which they cleaned their teeth.

Another factor which may have a bearing upon dental health is the age of the tooth brush which is used in brushing the teeth. The survey indicated that the majority of persons interviewed used a toothbrush less than 6 months old (76%).

TABLE 13.6
Length of Time Present Toothbrush is in Use

Length of time present toothbrush is in use	Adults with some natural teeth											
	16–24		25–34		35–44		45–54		55+		All ages	
	M	F	M	F	M	F	M	F	M	F	M	F
	%	%	%	%	%	%	%	%	%	%	%	%
Less than 3 months . .	46	61	43	50	47	52	49	63	42	36	45	53
3 months but less than 6 months	28	27	25	33	27	25	27	20	26	30	26	27
6 months but less than 1 year .	8	10	19	13	9	21	10	10	17	16	13	14
1 year or more . . .	10	2	13	3	9	1	10	5	10	17	11	5
Don't know . . .	7	—	—	1	7	1	2	2	3	—	4	1
No toothbrush . .	1	—	—	—	1	—	2	—	2	1	1	—
BASES	88	93	86	98	75	87	59	59	59	64	367	401*

*Those who never cleaned their teeth were not asked about toothbrushes.

Not all persons who clean their teeth use toothpowder or toothpaste. Table 13.7 shows the very small percentage of persons using different materials for tooth cleaning.

Considerable advertising of toothpastes containing fluoride has taken place in recent years. Informants were asked whether or not the toothpaste they used contained fluoride. The interviewers were instructed that informants were not to check the toothpaste in use before answering the question. A fairly high figure of informants did know whether their toothpaste contained fluoride and this is taken as being due to advertising by the toothpaste manufacturers.

There is much less advertising of dental floss and of wood sticks used in gum stimulation. Such dental aids are usually used under the direction and advice of a dentist or dental hygienist. This is reflected in Tables 13.8 and 13.9.

TABLE 13.7
Tooth Cleaning Materials

Material used in tooth cleaning	Adults with some natural teeth											
	16–24		25–34		35–44		45–54		55+		All ages	
	M	F	M	F	M	F	M	F	M	F	M	F
	%	%	%	%	%	%	%	%	%	%	%	%
Toothpaste	100	99	98	100	99	100	91	97	96	98	97	99
Toothpowder	—	1	1	—	1	—	5	3	4	—	2	1
Something else . . .	—	—	1	—	—	—	4	—	—	2	1	—
BASE	87	93	86	98	75	87	59	59	59	64	367	401

TABLE 13.8
Fluoride and Non-Fluoride Toothpastes

Toothpaste used in tooth cleaning	Adults with some natural teeth											
	16–24		25–34		35–44		45–54		55+		All ages	
	M	F	M	F	M	F	M	F	M	F	M	F
	%	%	%	%	%	%	%	%	%	%	%	%
Contains fluoride . . .	83	81	79	81	60	75	60	63	66	48	71	72
Does not	2	5	3	7	13	9	19	10	7	9	8	8
Don't know . . .	15	14	18	12	27	16	21	27	27	41	21	20
TOTAL	100		100		100		100		100		100	
BASE	87	93	85	98	75	87	57	57	56	63	360	398

TABLE 13.9
Use of Dental Floss and Woodsticks

	16–24		25–34		35–44		45–54		55+		All ages	
	M	F	M	F	M	F	M	F	M	F	M	F
	%	%	%	%	%	%	%	%	%	%	%	%
Dental floss	2	8	1	5	3	4	2	5	—	4	2	5
Woodsticks . . .	6	1	6	5	4	11	5	14	2	2	5	6
Other	1	2	5	3	4	2	—	—	9	1	3	2
Do not use any of these . .	91	89	88	87	89	83	93	81	91	93	90	87
TOTAL	100		100		100		100		100		100	
BASE	88	93	86	98	75	87	59	59	59	64	367	401

Adults with some natural teeth (spanning column header)

The survey investigated the number of people who had been shown by the dentist how best to clean their teeth. The great majority (82%) said they had not been shown. Of the 18% who had been shown 84% said they had been shown by the dentist and 16% had been shown by a dental nurse or hygienist. Since the regular dental attenders are much more often in contact with the dentist, and have therefore had a much greater opportunity of being shown how best to clean their teeth, we might expect regular attenders to have been shown how best to clean their teeth more than the irregular or occasional attenders. More of the regular dental attenders said they had in fact been shown (Table 13.10). 25% of the regular attenders said they had been shown how to clean their teeth compared to just over 11% of those who only went to the dentist when having trouble. The fact remains however that those who had been given advice were only 18% of the total.

TABLE 13.10
Whether Shown How Best to Clean Teeth, by Dental Attendance Pattern

Whether shown how best to clean natural teeth	Regular check-up	Occasional check-up	Only when having trouble	All
	%	%	%	%
Given advice	25	21	11	18
Leaflet, poster, film	—	—	1	—
Not given advice	75	79	88	82
BASE—adults who clean their natural teeth .	298	98	387	783

Adult with some natural teeth (spanning column header)

Base numbers re-weighted.

TABLE 13.10A
The Difference Between Regular Attenders and Occasional Attenders of those Shown How Best to Clean Teeth by Dental Attendance Pattern

Whether shown how best to clean natural teeth	Regular check-up	Occasional check-up	Only when having trouble	All
	%	%	%	%
Dentist	82	90	84	84
Dental Nurse	18	10	16	16
BASES	76	20	45	141*

Adults with some natural teeth (spanning column header)

*Only 141 were actually given advice and so asked who gave them the advice.

13.3 Tooth Cleaning and Dental Health

The frequency and method of brushing the teeth seems to differ widely for different people, and next investigated was whether tooth brushing appears to be related to the person's dental health.

Tooth brushing seems to be associated with other dental behaviour (the frequency and method of tooth brushing is seen to vary with dental attendance), and it is therefore very difficult to single out the effect of tooth brushing. The only way to do this objectively is, of course, to set up an experimental situation in order to isolate and test the effect of tooth brushing alone. There are some points, however, which the survey data can illuminate. Three aspects of dental health which are of particular value to study in relation to tooth brushing are tooth decay, oral hygiene and gum trouble.

It should be possible to relate toothbrushing to total decay experience. Unfortunately survey data among adults raises two major obstacles. Firstly the tooth brushing information collected referred to the current habits of the person concerned whereas decay experience had built up over his lifetime. Secondly total decay experience among adults cannot be assumed to be the sum of the teeth that are filled, currently decayed or missing, since extracted teeth were not necessarily previously decayed. An estimate of decay experience among adults is therefore difficult (if not impossible) to make from the survey data.

When attempting to estimate current decay rather than decay experience the length of time since the last dental treatment was received becomes important. A person who visits the dentist in pain may receive emergency treatment to relieve the pain without having any other treatment. Therefore the only fairly homogeneous group is the regular attenders who have been to the dentist within a specified period. The study of tooth brushing and current decay was thus confined to those regular attenders who had visited the dentist in the six months prior to the survey (Table 13.11).

Among this group of regular attenders there was in fact some evidence that current decay was associated with the frequency of tooth brushing. Among those who brushed their teeth only once a day the proportion who were decay-free was lower than the proportion decay-free among those who brushed their teeth three or more times a day (59% and 78% respectively).

TABLE 13.11

The Number of Decayed Teeth Among Regular Attenders Who Have Been to the Dentist in the Six Months prior to Survey, by Frequency of Tooth Cleaning

Number of decayed teeth	Adults with some natural teeth, who go to the dentist for a regular check-up, and who have been to the dentist in the six months prior to survey†					
	Frequency of cleaning natural teeth					
	Never*	Less than daily	Once daily	Twice daily	Three or more times daily	All
	%	%	%	%	%	%
0	—	50	59	60	78	63
1–2	—	50	29	33	19	29
3–5	—	0	12	7	3	8
6 or more	—	0	0	0	0	0
	—	100	100	100	100	100
Average number of decayed teeth	—	0.5	0.8	0.7	0.3	0.6
BASES	—	2	42	98	32	174

Base numbers re-weighted.

*None of the "never" cleaners had attended a dentist within the previous six months.

†Table refers to those dentate adults who were examined.

The regular attenders who have visited the dentist in the six months prior to the survey are, of course, only a small proportion of all people with some natural teeth. For the majority of adults with some natural teeth an analysis of tooth brushing and current decay is less than meaningful. Clearly the subject of tooth cleaning and tooth decay is not one which can be tackled very satisfactorily from survey data.

The survey also investigated whether current toothbrushing habits are associated with current oral hygiene and gum condition. It is worth considering the extent to which toothbrushing could be associated with oral hygiene and gum conditions.

The dental examination provided a measure of current debris. Debris is built up in the short term and can be removed by toothbrushing. It should be possible therefore to establish a link between toothbrushing and debris.

Although calculus deposits, once formed, will need dental attention for their removal, it is feasible that adequate toothbrushing may prevent the formation of calculus in the first place. When considering the association, account should be taken of the likelihood of recent dental intervention.

TABLE 13.12

Oral Hygiene and Gum Condition by Frequency of Tooth Cleaning

	Adults with some natural teeth				
	Frequency of cleaning natural teeth				
	Less than daily	Once daily	Twice daily	Three or more times daily	All
	%	%	%	%	%
DEBRIS					
Zero	67	79	83	81	80
One	33	21	17	19	20
	100	100	100	100	100
CALCULUS					
Zero	33	44	56	43	42
One	67	56	44	57	58
	100	100	100	100	100
GINGIVITIS					
Zero	100	90	99	100	97
One	0	0	0	0	0
Two	0	10	1	0	3
	100	100	100	100	100
PERIODONTAL					
Zero	92	85	94	100	92
One	8	15	6	0	8
	100	100	100	100	100
Overall average					
BASES	16	68	138	42	264

Base numbers re-weighted.

Toothbrushing is recommended as a method of reducing and preventing the milder levels of gum disease and therefore toothbrushing could be of interest in relation to the gum condition. There are complications however, since a dentist may have suggested to a patient that, because of the state of the patient's gums the patient's toothbrushing habits need to be altered in order to improve the health of the gums.

In such cases the implied cause and effect relationship is reversed, and the associations may be completely masked. Thus, cause and effect cannot be measured by survey data, but only by a properly designed experiment.

Table 13.12 gives the level of oral hygiene and the periodontal condition in relation to the frequency of toothbrushing, for all adults with some natural teeth, and we consider firstly the situation with regard to debris, given in the first section of the table.

It could be expected that regular tooth cleaning would reduce the amount of debris on the teeth. Such would appear to be the case. Persons who clean their teeth twice per day or more have a greater proportion of zero debris scores than those who clean their teeth less frequently.

It would be logical to assume also that a lower incidence of calculus, healthier gingival and improved periodontal health would result from regular toothbrushing. The England and Wales and the Scotland surveys indicated that there was such a relationship. In the Northern Ireland survey there was a higher proportion of zero periodontal scores among those who brush their teeth regularly. Although 55% of dentate adults clean their teeth at least twice per day and although 76% used a toothbrush less than six months old, there was little difference between regular and irregular brushers in relation to zero gingivitis scores. A further study of the methods of toothbrushing rather than the frequency of toothbrushing might provide interesting information. 82% of informants with natural teeth had not been given advice on how best to clean their teeth (Table 13.10). This total compares with the 84% in the Scotland survey who were not shown how best to clean their teeth.

14. Public Attitudes to the Appearance of the Teeth

14.1 Orthodontic Treatment

One aspect of dental treatment which is of interest to the responsible authorities is that of orthodontic treatment, the correction of irregularities in the teeth. Although there seems to be increased awareness of the benefits to be gained from the correction of such irregularities it is difficult to gauge the public attitudes towards orthodontic treatment and its benefits in terms of speech, mastication and dental health as well as appearance. The importance of having teeth straightened in relation to both adults and children was investigated. Adults' perception of their own appearance plays a part in their attitude to corrective treatment for their children and the survey attempted to establish the attitude of adults to having teeth straightened.

Adults considered that the straightening of children's crooked or protruding teeth was very important (79%) with (17%) considering it fairly important. 3% considered it not very important and 1% not at all important.

57% of adults considered the straightening of adult's teeth to be very important, 24% fairly important and 16% not very important, 3% considered it not at all important.

14.2 Satisfaction with the Appearance of the Natural Teeth

Informants were asked if they were satisfied with the appearance of their natural teeth. 76% said that they were satisfied and 24% said they were dissatisfied. Persons who said that they were dissatisfied with the appearance of their teeth were asked about the aspects of the appearance of their teeth which caused them dissatisfaction. The results are shown in Table 14.1.

TABLE 14.1

Aspects of the Appearance of the Teeth which Caused Dissatisfaction

	Male	Female
	%	%
Crooked, Protruding	34	38
Gaps, space between teeth	10	14
Size/shape of teeth	13	7
Broken/chipped teeth	10	4
Colour	13	19
Fillings	5	7
Decayed/Bad	14	7
Other	1	4
TOTAL	100	100
BASE	69	117

14.3 Discussion of the Appearance of the Teeth with the Dentist

The survey further asked persons who were dissatisfied with the appearance of their teeth if they had ever talked to a dentist about it. 38% had talked to a dentist and 62% had not. Those who had talked to a dentist were asked to provide information on what the dentist said while those who had not talked to a dentist were asked to give reasons why they had not discussed their feelings with the dentist. The results are given in Tables 14.2 and 14.3.

79

TABLE 14.2

Dentists Comments on Informants' Dissatisfaction with the Appearance of their Teeth

	Male	Female
	%	%
Dentist will treat it	33	23
Advised against treatment	27	26
Nothing can be done	27	36
Teeth are all right, nothing to worry about .	13	9
Other	—	6
BASE	15	47*

*Very few who were not satisfied with their teeth actually spoke to the dentist.

TABLE 14.3

Informants' Reasons for Not Discussing Appearance of the Teeth with a Dentist

	Male	Female
	%	%
No reason	55	42
Fear of dentist	7	14
Never go to the dentist	26	16
Dentist won't be able to do anything . .	4	13
Not really worried about it . . .	2	5
No opportunity to talk/I am always in a hurry .	6	5
Other	—	5
TOTAL	100	100
BASE	47	57*

*Very few who were not satisfied with their teeth actually spoke to the dentist.

Some relationship may exist between the appearance of the natural teeth and the importance attached to wearing a denture for appearance rather than utility.

14.4   Appearance and the Denture Wearer

Denture wearers were asked whether their first false teeth were mainly for the sake of appearance or mainly to help them eat. 69% said that the dentures were mainly for the sake of appearance and 26% said that they were mainly for eating; 5% said they were for both reasons.

15. Knowledge about Factors which affect the Natural Teeth; Dental Attendance and Dental Fitness

In this chapter three separate lines of enquiry about dental health are pursued. Firstly the variation in knowledge about factors which affect dental health; secondly the sub-groups of the dentate population most likely to have established a pattern of regular dental attendance, and thirdly the proportion of dentate adults found to be dentally fit at the time of the survey examination.

15.1 Factors which affect Dental Health

During the interview questions were asked about factors for keeping teeth healthy. The factors that we asked about were:—

  (i) not eating sweets;
 (ii) regular visits to the dentist;
(iii) cleaning teeth regularly;
(iv) having fluoride in the water;
 (v) adding fluoride to the water.

Informants were asked to categorise the factors as very important, fairly important, not very important or not at all important.

Factors which were fairly commonly known were chosen and therefore 'acceptable' answers rather than true personal opinions could be expected. This did not negate the usefulness of the question. The level of 'acceptable' answers varied between different people, and the level of importance ascribed to the different factors relative to each other was investigated. The results are given in Table 15.1, in the order in which the factors appeared in the question.

The relative position of the five factors is first examined. 86% of adults said that regular tooth cleaning was very important for keeping teeth healthy, 70% said that regular visits to the dentist were very important, 52% said that not eating sweets was very important, 21% said that having fluoride in the water and 23% said that adding fluoride to the water was very important for keeping teeth healthy. It is interesting to find that tooth cleaning is nearly universally accepted as being very important for dental health. It is the translation of the idea into practice which is more difficult to attain universally (see Chapter 13).

The survey investigated whether men and women differed in the proportions who thought the various factors to be very important. A higher proportion of women than men said dental attendance and tooth cleaning were very important.

Not eating sweets was considered a very important factor in keeping the teeth healthy by a smaller proportion of people than either regular visits to the dentist or cleaning the teeth regularly.

There is an overall similarity between the ratings of the five factors. For example although irregular dental attenders were less likely to say that regular dental visits were important than were the regular attenders, nevertheless 68% of them did say it was very important. Similarly 87% of irregular dental attenders considered that regular tooth cleaning was very important. It would seem that it is not so much within basic knowledge that the problem of improving dental health lies but in the motivation of people to act upon the knowledge that they have.

TABLE 15.1

Proportion of People considering each Factor to be Very Important in Keeping Teeth Healthy

Proportion considering each factor to be very important in keeping teeth healthy	Not eating sweets %	Regular visits to the dentist %	Cleaning teeth regularly %	Having fluoride in the water* ·%	Adding fluoride to the water* %	BASES
All adults	52	70	86	21	23	1,176
Men	48	65	79	22	24	536
Women	55	74	91	20	22	640
Edentulous adults . .	53	62	79	18	19	393
Dentate adults . . .	51	74	89	22	25	783
Dentate adults:—‡						
Regular attenders . .	55	89	95	24	27	325
Occasional attenders .	43	68	87	16	21	128
Only when have trouble.	52	61	81	19	21	704
Social class:—†						
I, II and III non-manual	50	73	89	19	20	318
III manual . . .	49	70	86	22	26	226
IV and V . . .	55	66	78	15	19	216
Housewife . . .	56	74	89	25	29	283
Age:—						
16–24	46	78	92	25	28	185
25–34	48	70	89	25	28	191
35–44	59	77	91	23	26	191
45–54	55	75	86	15	21	179
55 and over . . .	51	61	79	18	18	430

Base numbers re-weighted.
*There was a high number of "don't knows" in this section.
†Students, non-classifiables, refusals etc. not included.
‡Does not include those who never attend.

15.2 Who are the Regular Dental Attenders?

Throughout the report it has been shown that people's stated dental attendance pattern has a significant relationship with their dental health. Sometimes it has not been obvious whether the benefit of regular attendance has accrued as a result of direct dentist intervention, or whether the attitudes which made the individual a regular attender are the more important factors.

It may well be the attitudes which cause a person to be regular attender which are important. In that case it will not be enough to change dental attendance patterns alone if attitudes towards restorative treatment, personal oral hygiene, and the acceptability of dentures do not change, and therefore remain out of line with the current attitudes of regular attenders.

The discussion of attendance patterns is confined to dentate adults since the dental care required for full dentures is of a completely different nature.

TABLE 15.2

Dental Attendance Pattern for Adults of Different Ages with Some Natural Teeth

Attendance pattern	Adults with some natural teeth					
	Present age					All ages
	16–24	25–34	35–44	45–54	55 and over	
	%	%	%	%	%	%
Regular check-up . .	45	29	42	29	13	28
Occasional check-up . .	14	18	12	10	6	11
Only when having trouble .	41	53	46	61	81	61
	100	100	100	100	100	100
BASES	183	191	190	177	435	1,176

Base numbers re-weighted.

Table 15.2 shows, for those with some natural teeth, how dental attendance varied with age. The variation was not very marked: a fairly constant proportion of people in each age group went to the dentist for a regular check-up, but there was an increase with age in the proportion who only went when they were having trouble. It is of particular interest to examine the two youngest age groups, that is those aged 16–24 and those aged 25–34. Even among these people, about one third were in the habit of going to the dentist for a regular check-up, and almost half only went when they were having trouble with their teeth.

The dental attendance patterns of men and women were rather different, as is shown in Table 15.3. A greater proportion of women said they went to the dentist for a regular check-up than men (31% compared to 24%) and, conversely, a greater proportion of men went only when they were having trouble (66% compared to 57% for women).

TABLE 15.3

Dental Attendance Pattern for Different Sexes

Attendance pattern	Adults with some natural teeth		
	Males	Females	Both sexes
	%	%	%
Regular check-up .	24	31	28
Occasional check-up .	10	12	11
Only when having trouble .	66	57	61
	100	100	100
BASES .	536	640	1,176

Base numbers re-weighted.

Dental attendance pattern also varied greatly with social class (Table 15.4), those people in the top social class group being markedly different from other people. In this top group 41% of adults with some natural teeth were in the habit of going to the dentist for a regular check-up, compared to only 18% in the lowest social class group. Among adults in the highest social class group 48% went only when they were having trouble compared with 68% in the lowest social class group (the proportion of people who went for an occasional check-up was fairly constant for all social classes).

TABLE 15.4

Dental Attendance Pattern, for Adults of Different Social Classes

Attendance pattern	Adults with some natural teeth				
	I, II and III non-manual	III manual	IV non-manual, IV manual and V	Housewife	All social classes
	%	%	%	%	%
Regular check-up .	41	26	18	23	28
Occasional check-up .	11	11	14	10	11
Only when having trouble .	48	63	68	67	61
	100	100	100	100	100
BASES . .	381	226	222	289	1,176

Base numbers re-weighted.

It would therefore appear that among those with some natural teeth, dental attendance varies with sex, social class, and age.

Anyone wishing to improve regular dental attendance would need to direct their attention to females in the lower social class groups and males of any social class group. The difference in the proportions of regular attenders among the females in the different social class groups suggests that women might be easier to convert to regular attendance and that a special approach might be needed for the men.

15.3 How Many Dentate Adults Are Dentally Fit?

Among adults who still had some natural teeth at the time of the survey there was considerable variation from person to person as to how many natural teeth were still present. The chance of having any active decay, or being involved periodontally at the time of the survey was to some extent dependent on the number of teeth at risk. The findings on dental fitness for several different groups defined by their previous tooth loss and denture provision are presented.

People who had no currently decayed teeth and no contra-indication with respect to gum condition were designated dentally fit. This was a fairly harsh definition in so far as it includes debris, calculus, gingivitis and periodontitis as contra-indications, and perhaps the dentist himself cannot be expected to be responsible for attaining this level of patient dental fitness; but the dentist and patient should, together, be aiming at this level.

Since the different component parts of estimates of the person's gum condition play varying roles of importance their contributions are shown separately as well as in combination (Table 15.6).

Among all dentate adults 43% had no active decay at the time of the survey. There was some difference in the rates of no active decay according to the numbers of teeth at risk. The greatest difference was seen in the group who had lost twelve or more teeth but had not been provided with any dentures, among whom fewer than one in three were decay-free at the time of the survey. The fact that extensive tooth loss had not resulted in the provision of dentures suggests that these were not particularly dentally-conscious people.

As far as the presence of debris was concerned the only group that differed were the people with a full upper denture, for whom a higher proportion of debris-free mouths were found. Here again, of course, the complete absence of teeth in the upper jaw (and maybe extensive loss in the lower jaw as well) reduced the risk of finding debris on natural teeth.

TABLE 15.6

Proportion of Dentate Adults Dentally Fit, showing Variations in Risk

| Proportion with: | Adults with some natural teeth | | | | | |
| | No dentures | | | Dentures | | |
	5 or fewer teeth missing	6–11 teeth missing	12 or more teeth missing	Not a full upper denture	Full upper denture	All
	%	%	%	%	%	%
No decay . . .	52	44	31	35	49	43
No debris . . .	84	82	73	70	79	79
No calculus . .	50	40	32	40	37	42
No gingivitis . .	73	71	57	57	60	67
No periodontitis . .	93	91	79	75	79	86
No gum trouble at all .	42	33	21	26	30	32
No decay nor gum trouble (ie "dentally fit") . .	27	16	9	11	16	17
BASES . . .	161	196	68	124	43	592

Base numbers re-weighted.

The presence of calculus varied with the number of teeth at risk, the highest proportion of calculus-free people being found amongst those with the least number of missing teeth. This association reflects the fact that age is very much associated with tooth loss and that the group of people with five or fewer missing natural teeth are more likely to be calculus-free because they are younger, age offsetting the fact that they have more teeth at risk. It is in fact those with no dentures and the greatest tooth loss who have the least proportion (32%) calculus-free, this group again being affected by age.

The proportion of people with no gum trouble at all is 32%. If one combines both healthy gum condition and freedom from current decay, then one arrives at the proportion of dentate adults found to be dentally fit. Of all dentate adults this proved to be 17%; among those who had lost five or fewer natural teeth it was 27%. If one defines being dentally fit as being without gum inflammation and without decay, few dentate adults are achieving dental fitness.

15.4 Expense of Dental Treatment

Attitudes to dental treatment can have an effect on dental health. In Chapter 14 public attitudes to the appearance of the teeth were discussed and whether they had discussed the appearance with their dentists. Public attitudes to dental treatment can possibly be affected by costs. 21% of persons visiting the dentist normally have some idea of how much the treatment is going to cost but 79% do not. 21% knew where they could obtain information about Health Service dental charges but 79% did not.

The majority of dentists, (66%) did not usually tell patients how the total cost of dental treatment is made up. In order to assess the accuracy of public knowledge about the costs of dental treatment, a list of the commoner items of dental treatment was presented. Estimates were made of whether each course of treatment would cost £2.00 or less, between £2.00 and £5.00 or more.

TABLE 15.7
Estimated Costs of Dental Treatment

	Free	£2.00 or less	Between £2.00 and £5.00	£5.00 or more	Don't know
	%	%	%	%	%
Exam. 2 extractions	1	5	22	29	43
Exam. 1 large filling, 1 extraction . .	1	6	22	26	45
Examination only	23	22	6	4	45
Exam. 2 X-rays, scale and polish, 1 small filling	1	7	16	28	48
Exam. 4 extractions, new dentures fitted .	0.5	0.5	2	51	46
Exam. 2 X-rays, 6 extractions, gen. anaesthetic	0.5	0.5	4	46	49
Repair of cracked denture	4	9	13	17	57
Exam. 2 X-rays, scale and polish . . .	1	9	18	22	50

33% of persons thought that the £7.00 which was the patients portion of the Health Service dental treatment fee was too high, 64% about right and 3% too low.

41% knew what kinds of treatment cost the patient more than the standard portion.

72% knew the kinds of people who are entitled to free treatment, 49% specified expectant or nursing mothers and 51% specified others such as:—

(1) Low income/Supplement benefit/FIS   15%

(2) Old age pensioners   14%

(3) Other including National Assistance, other Govt. aid   22%

16% of full denture wearers said that they knew the current charge to the patient of a full set of Health Service dentures (£36.00). They were asked how much:—

71% said £30.00

11% said £20.00—£30.00

5% said £10.00–£20.00

The remaining 13% gave various other answers.

15.5 Denture Acceptance

If there is general acceptance of the wearing of dentures the care of the natural teeth of the population may suffer.

Chapter 12 discussed extractions and dentures and the attitudes towards partial and full dentures. The informants provided further information about their attitudes to the inevitability of full dentures. 31% considered that at some time they would have to have full dentures; 57% that they would keep their natural teeth and 12% did not know.

15% of persons thought that all or most of the persons they knew of similar age to themselves had full dentures, 31% thought that some of them had, 53 % very few or none of them and 1% did not know.

15.6 Sweets and Sugars

The part which sugars play in dental disease is well known to the dental profession and to other health professions. What is less well known is how widely the knowledge is spread throughout the community.

It is also not known how much advice dentists or dental staff give to the public on sugars or foods which contain sugars. 12% stated that they had been advised about eating sweets and other sugary foods but 88% had not. The advice was given by a dentist in 84% of the cases, a dental nurse of hygienist in 14% and by somebody else in 2% of the cases. These findings support the results shown in Table 15.1.

16. Early Tooth Loss Among Women

One curious anomaly which was established in the England and Wales survey of 1968 was that when asked about their attitudes towards dentistry, their attendance patterns and their dental habits, women seemed to be more dentally aware and have better dental habits than men. Yet it was women who, in the younger age groups, appeared to be the first to lose all their natural teeth.

There seemed to be a larger concentration of the incidence of total tooth loss coinciding with child-bearing and the years thereafter. The linking of child-bearing and total tooth loss may have been encouraged by the dental regulations of the Health Service. In 1948 when the Health Service began, all dental treatment was free to the patient. Subsequently, charges to the patient were introduced but priority classes could continue to obtain free treatment, and one of these priority classes was that of pregnant and nursing mothers. It is possible that there was a link between free treatment and early tooth loss. It is notable however that the discrepancy between tooth loss in men and women in the UK has lessened since the 1968 England and Wales survey. At that time in the 35–44 age group 28% of women had lost all their teeth compared with 16.3% of men. The lessening may reflect an increased awareness of dental health. The first part of the UK report* indicates changing patterns of dental care between 1968 and 1978 and it is possible that more women prefer to retain their natural teeth now than formerly.

Persons interviewed in the Northern Ireland survey who had no natural teeth of their own were asked at what age they had had their remaining natural teeth extracted. Those persons who had had all their remaining teeth extracted before the age of thirty were identified. Table 16.1 gives the current age group of these persons.

The older age groups tend to have a higher proportion of persons who were edentulous before the age of thirty. The table indicates that a smaller proportion of persons under thirty is being rendered edentulous among the younger age groups.

The link between free treatment and edentulousness is not clear. Although there is a higher proportion of women than men who have lost all their teeth by the age of thirty in the two youngest age groups, the pattern is reversed in the older age groups. The link between free treatment and edentulousness cannot be shown in either of the groups of women who would have been of child-bearing age in the years following 1948.

In persons under 45, there is a tendency for more women to lose all their teeth than is the case for men (Table 16.2). Gum disease seems to be a common cause of tooth loss among younger men than among women. It is not however possible to ascribe the higher proportion of tooth loss among younger women to either dental decay or gum disease.

TABLE 16.1

Persons Rendered Edentulous Before the Age of Thirty

Current age	Male	Female	All
	%	%	%
30–34	3	5	4
35–44	13	19	17
45–54	20	17	18
55–64	23	21	22
65–75	34	19	24
75+	7	19	15
	100	100	100

---

*Adult Dental Health (Vol. 1) England and Wales 1968–1978. J. E. Todd and A. M. Walker. HMSO 1980.

TABLE 16.2
Reasons for the Extraction of the Remaining Natural Teeth

Current age	Male		Female		All	
	Decay	Gum disease	Decay	Gum disease	Decay	Gum disease
30–34	0	7	5	5	4	5
35–44	7	22	19	19	16	15
45–54	21	14	16	19	18	13
55–64	29	21	19	24	22	18
65–75	29	36	22	14	22	40
75+	14	0	19	19	18	9
	100	100	100	100	100	100

17.   The Experience of Dental Treatment

A pleasant experience can produce the desire to undergo a similar experience on a later occasion. Similarly an unpleasant experience can produce the determination not to undergo such an experience again. Because of the possible bearing on attitudes to dental health, the survey investigated previous dental experiences.

17.1   Childhood Dental Experiences

Thirty-four per cent of persons were given a great deal of encouragement to clean their teeth, 30% a fair amount and 23% were not given much encouragement, whilst 13% were given no encouragement at all.

Most persons (70%) had visited a dentist when they were children, that is before the age of 16 but a proportion (30%) had not.

Of those who had visited the dentist 37% went to a school dentist, 49% to some other dentist and 14% to both. Those children who went to other dentists or to both the school dentist and some other dentist went for a regular check up (34%), an occasional check up (16%) or only when having trouble with their teeth (50%).

Fifty-four per cent had had teeth filled before the age of 16 and 39% had not. Seven per cent could not remember.

Sixty-seven per cent had had teeth extracted, 26% had not and 7% could not remember.

Eight per cent had been given treatment to straighten their teeth, either by means of a brace (orthodontic appliance) or by extractions, but 92% had not.

Sixty-one per cent of those who had been given treatment to straighten the teeth had worn a brace, 20% had had extractions, 13% had both and 6% had other treatment.

17.2   Adult Dental Experiences

Sixty-eight per cent of persons had had fillings as an adult but 32% had not. Of those persons who had teeth filled 82% had an injection in the gum and 18% did not.

The advent of intravenous anaesthesia in dentistry is reflected in the 4% of persons who had been given an injection in the arm to kill the pain of a filling.

Seventy-seven per cent of persons usually have an injection of some sort for fillings. Ninety-three per cent of persons had experienced extractions as an adult. 49% had experienced gas (a general anaesthetic), 78% a local anaesthetic (injection in the gum) and 7% an intravenous anaesthetic (injection in the arm) for extraction.

17.3   X-Ray Experience

Thirty-seven per cent of persons had had an X-ray of the teeth taken. Fifteen per cent usually have an X-ray when visiting the dentist and 85% do not.

17.4   Wisdom Teeth

Because the last permanent molar teeth commonly called the wisdom teeth are the last teeth to erupt and erupt in adult life, they are usually noticed and remembered. Information was sought on each tooth and on whether informants thought that the tooth was still standing or had been removed.

TABLE 17.1

Wisdom Teeth

	Upper left	Upper right	Upper left	Upper right
	%	%	%	%
Wisdom tooth has come through . . .	70	69	69	69
Wisdom tooth has not come through . .	11	12	12	13
Don't know	19	19	19	18
Wisdom tooth still standing . . .	62	63	61	63
Wisdom tooth has been taken out . . .	38	37	39	37

17.5 Most Recent Visit to the Dentist

Fifty-four per cent of persons last visited the dentist because they had been having trouble with their teeth, 43% for a check up and 3% for some other reason.

Those who had last visited the dentist because they were having trouble with their teeth went because of toothache 84%, fillings 7%, broken teeth 6%, other 3%.

Forty-six per cent had made one visit, 23% two visits, 14% three visits, 9% four visits and 8% five or more visits on the last occasion that they had consulted the dentist.

During the last course of treatment many persons experienced a variety of items of dental care. The results are shown in Table 17.2.

TABLE 17.2

Last Course of Dental Treatment

	Yes	No
	%	%
X-rays taken . . .	13	87
Teeth filled . . .	43	57
Teeth extracted . . .	40	60
Teeth scaled . . .	41	59

17.6 Costs of Dental Treatment

Experience of dental costs could have an affect on patterns of dental care. Informants were asked how much their last course of dental treatment had cost. Thirty-seven per cent said that it had cost less than £5.00, 38% between £5.00 and £7.00 and 5% between £7.00 and £10.00. Twenty per cent had cost more than £10.00. Twenty-three per cent said that this was more than they expected, 61% about what they expected, 14% less than expected and 2% thought something else. Some persons had not paid anything for their dental treatment. Of these, 50% were under 21, were pregnant or the mother of a child under one year old, 15% received remission of charges on the grounds of low income and 18% for other reasons such as that no treatment was necessary. Eighty-five per cent had expected the treatment to be free.

17.7 Availability of Health Service Treatment

In the 5 years previous to the survey 4% of persons had difficulty in obtaining Health Service dental treatment, 86% had no difficulty and 10% had not tried to obtain treatment.

Of those who had difficulty in obtaining Health Service treatment, 19% had difficulty in obtaining it at all and 50% had difficulty in obtaining extractions. The other 31% had difficulty in obtaining fillings, dentures or crowns. When asked what they did about it 35% said that they went privately, 30% did nothing and the others searched around for another dentist.

17.8 Persons Who Do Not Attend the Dentist Regularly

In previous chapters attention has been paid to dental attendance patterns, to regular attenders for dental examinations, and to non-attenders.

In general 28% of persons attend for a regular check up, 11% for an occasional check up and 61% only when having trouble. The main reasons given for not attending regularly for examination were:—

1. Apathetic, too lazy   32%
2. Had not had any trouble   18%
3. Afraid   17%

Information was sought on the circumstances under which the non-regular attenders would visit the dentist. The results are shown in Table 17.3.

TABLE 17.3

Circumstances under which Non-Attenders Would Visit the Dentist

	Yes	No
	%	%
Occasional twinges of toothache . . .	44	56
A tooth which felt loose	51	49
Not been to the dentist for a long time . .	25	75
A swollen face	61	39
Sore gums	52	48
Toothache causing wakefulness all night . .	94	6
A gumboil	48	52
A tooth with a piece broken off . .	46	54
Gums which bled occasionally	30	70

Eighteen per cent of persons stated that they currently attended the dentist more often than 5 years before the survey, 56% about the same and 26% less often.

The main reasons for going less often were:—

1. Have no/less trouble with the teeth 30%
2. Fewer teeth left   25%
3. Can't be bothered   12%

17.9   Reasons for Non-attendance

There are several reasons why people do not attend the dentist. The most common reasons were listed for the survey and those which applied to informants were identified. The results are shown in Table 17.4.

TABLE 17.4

Reasons for Non-Attendance for Dental Treatment

Put off going to the dentist because:	APPLIES				
	Very much	A fair amount	Not much	Not at all	Don't know
	%	%	%	%	%
I'm scared of the dentist . . .	15	10	14	60	1
It's difficult to get time off work . .	6	8	8	76	2
I don't like having fillings . . .	16	14	23	45	2
It's too expensive to go too often . .	13	10	12	62	3
I haven't got a regular dentist . .	12	5	5	76	2
I can't be bothered really . . .	16	12	11	59	2
I don't like the thought of having teeth out .	18	11	18	52	1
It's difficult to get an appointment . .	7	11	11	69	2
It's a long way to go	3	4	8	81	4

Of the 65% who found something unpleasant about visiting the dentist, the most unpleasant aspects of a visit to the dentist were:—

1. Filling/drilling/noise of the drill   23%
2. Injections   20%
3. Waiting   18%
4. Apprehension   13%

18. The Dental Health of Adults in Northern Ireland— A Summary

Dental surveys of the kind carried out in 1979 can be used to measure the prevalence of dental health and disease in the population at a particular time. In this case the time was six weeks in the Autumn of 1979. However useful the information and however interesting the results, they can only provide a snapshot view of dental health. Nevertheless the results of the survey provide a useful base of information, and give a body of knowledge previously unobtainable which should aid in the planning of dental services.

The information will become more useful if similar surveys are carried out in future years. The 1978 United Kingdom survey has provided patterns of the incidence of dental disease by comparing the results of that survey with those of the broadly similar surveys carried out in England and Wales in 1968 and in Scotland in 1972.

Because the Northern Ireland survey is the first to be carried out, local comparisons are not possible. Comparison with the results of the UK survey which used the same techniques and criteria should however provide interesting comparisons of dental health and attitudes in Northern Ireland with those of the rest of the United Kingdom.

18.1 Edentulousness as an Indicator of Dental Health

A useful indicator of dental health in a community is the proportion of adults with no natural teeth. In Northern Ireland 33% of the population were edentulous, with the highest proportions in the age groups above 55 years. The proportion in England and Wales who have lost all their teeth has fallen since the England and Wales survey of 1968 (37%) to 29% in 1978. It is to be hoped that a similar reduction in the proportion of totally edentulous persons will be found eventually in Northern Ireland. One hopeful indication may be that the proportion of edentulous persons in the under 30 age group is more like that of England and Wales than is the case with the groups between 35 and 65.

18.2 The Edentulous

We have seen (Table 4.1) that below the age of 65, a higher proportion of persons in Northern Ireland is edentulous than is the case in England and Wales. The proportion of edentulous people varies widely with class. The professional, managerial and non-manual skilled classes have a much lower proportion of edentulous persons (16%) than the manual semi-skilled and unskilled classes (47%). Most are female, married and over 55. Edentulous persons tend not to visit the dentist unless having trouble (85%). The majority of the edentulous (59%) have had no experience of restorative dental treatment.

18.3 Denture Wearers

Where all the teeth have been lost virtually everybody has been supplied with full dentures (94%). The vast majority (80%) wear both dentures all day. There is a high degree of satisfaction with the appearance of the dentures, 76% were very satisfied and 14% fairly satisfied with the appearance of their dentures.

18.4 Acceptance of Total Tooth Loss

Half of the denture wearers were either glad or untroubled at the loss of their natural teeth. Even among the regular attenders with natural teeth there was a substantial minority (12%) who did not feel at all upset at the prospect of losing all their teeth. Such a wide acceptance of total tooth loss among adults indicates the low priority given by a large section of the population to the retention of the natural teeth.

18.5 Patterns of Dental Care

As well as the status of dental health in the community, the survey was designed to obtain some information on the sort of dental care which was sought and received under the dental services. A useful indicator of dental care is the number of the teeth which have been filled but which are otherwise sound. The average number of filled, otherwise sound teeth in the Northern Ireland survey was 8.4 teeth. This compares favourably with the 7.8 filled but otherwise sound teeth found in England and Wales during the 1978 survey. The proportion of teeth filled but also decayed was similar in Northern Ireland, 0.6 teeth per person on average, and the 0.7 found in England and Wales. The decayed teeth showed similar proportions in Northern Ireland and in England and Wales, decayed but restorable averaged 0.9 and 0.7 teeth respectively and unrestorable 0.3 teeth in each case.

The main difference occurred in the average number of missing teeth. In Northern Ireland there was an average number of 10.1 teeth missing per mouth. As an adult mouth contains 32 teeth, this represents a 30% loss of the possible teeth. The average number of missing teeth in England and Wales was 8.8.

18.6 The Health of the Gums

Healthy gums are an important factor in the retention of permanent teeth by adults. The standards of gum health were high. 79% of adults with some natural teeth were recorded as having a zero total debris score. As the informants who were going to have a dental examination knew the date and time of the examination, it is possible that some of them had cleaned their teeth just prior to the dentists arrival. The other criteria for healthy gums however seem to indicate that there is a fairly high standard of gum health among adults in Northern Ireland. 42% of those examined had a total calculus score of zero and 67% had a total gingivitis score of zero. The proportion with a zero periodontitis score was 86%. It should be remembered however that gum disease is associated with the teeth. Where many teeth are missing, the amount of gum disease is likely to be less than when there are many teeth present. The measurement of gum health has been found to be among the least reliable measurements of dental health in dental surveys (Appendix 7). Results should be interpreted accordingly.

18.7 Dentists and Patients

There seems to be a high degree of continuity in the relationship between dentist and patient. 65% of informants have been attending their present dentist for 5 years or more. While nearness of the dental practice was given as the reason for choosing a particular dentist by 22% of the persons interviewed and recommendation for 30%, almost a quarter (22%) regarded their dentist as the family dentist. Although dentists contract to treat their patients only for a course of treatment and do not have a list or panel of patients in the way that general medical practitioners do, they are regarded in the same light by many of their patients. There does not seem to be any great difficulty in obtaining an appointment. 60% of informants were able to arrange an appointment within two weeks.

18.8 Private Treatment

It is always difficult to estimate the amount of private dental treatment carried out. Arrangements between dentists and patients for private treatment are not subject to Health Service regulations and therefore are not the responsibility of the Department or the Health and Social Services Boards. Yet the extent of private treatment could have a bearing upon the provision of dental services which are necessary to supply the needs of the population. For this reason an attempt was made to estimate the extent of private dental treatment. There is so little dental treatment provided privately that it is very difficult to draw any conclusions from the information provided by the very small sample of persons who had obtained private treatment. Perhaps surprisingly, a higher percentage of extractions and fillings (30% each) was provided privately than either crowns and bridges (20%) or dentures (10%). The preferences for private or health service treatment are not clear, but the main reasons for obtaining private dental treatment seem to be mainly a desire for better quality treatment (25%) or a wish for the treatment to be provided quickly (24%).

18.9 Availability of Health Service Dental Treatment

It would seem that there is no great difficulty in obtaining Health Service dental treatment. 75% of the persons interviewed described dental treatment as easy to obtain and 87% considered that dental services were convenient. However there can arise situations when there is urgent need for dental treatment. Only 4% of the persons interviewed had sought emergency dental treatment during the previous five years. Most (61%) expressed satisfaction at the promptness with which they had obtained emergency treatment. Most people (78%) considered that the general dental service was satisfactory. There is less knowledge about community dental services than about general dental services. 50% did not know or had no opinion about school dental services. 87% did not know or had no opinion about dental services to the handicapped. However as adults attend general dental practitioners rather than the other dental services, this is not surprising. What is rather surprising is the proportion who travel to the dental surgery by car or motor cycle (40%) although most people (51%) live within two miles of the dental surgery.

18.10 Preferences for Dental Treatment

Most people expressed a preference for fillings rather than the extraction of a back tooth (60% as against 38%) and also a front tooth (84% as against 15%). Persons under 55 tended to prefer fillings to extractions for back teeth but all age groups had a majority of persons in favour of fillings in front teeth. In general the higher social classes and the regular attenders preferred fillings to extractions.

18.11 Tooth Cleaning

The frequency of tooth cleaning seems to be associated with dental attendance patterns and with social class. Regular attenders for dental treatment and members of the higher social groups brush their teeth more frequently than the members of other groups.

18.12 Appearance of the Teeth

The appearance of the teeth is quite important in the minds of many adults. 79% of informants considered the straightening of children's crooked or protruding teeth to be very important and 69% of denture wearers had their first set of false teeth for the sake of appearance. Most people were satisfied with the appearance of their natural teeth. Those who were not, were most concerned by crooked or protruding teeth.

18.13 Factors which can affect Dental Health

In the younger age groups, there is a tendency for more women than men to lose all their teeth. It is not possible however to state whether dental decay or gum disease is the cause.

Most people had visited the dentist as a child (70%) and 68% had had fillings as an adult. Of the adult dental attenders 82% had a local anaesthetic for conservation. Health Service dental treatment was obtained without difficulty by 86% of people. Perhaps because of this there were more than twice as many persons who attended the dentist only when having trouble than regular attenders. The main reasons for the failure to attend was apathy (32%) but dislike of the commoner forms of dental treatment such as fillings and extractions were also expressed.

18.14 Dental Health and Dental Needs

From all the information gathered for the survey, it should be possible to describe the characteristics of dental health in Northern Ireland and to form a picture of the needs for dental care and the dental attitudes of the population.

It could be expected that the majority of persons in need of dental care will have fewer teeth than their counterparts in England and Wales. Edentulous persons are likely to be over 55 years, married and female with no history of restorative treatment. Most people will have healthy gums and will have attended the same dentist for more than 5 years. They have little experience of private treatment perhaps because most people find dental services easy and convenient to obtain, and are satisfied with the general dental services and with emergency treatment. Half live within two miles of the dental surgery. Most people would rather have their teeth filled than extracted, go to the dentist only when having trouble and have visited the dentist as children. As might be expected, the regular attenders of the higher social classes brush their teeth most frequently.

18.15 Conclusion

It would be inappropriate for a report such as this which has been prepared to provide information about dental health to make any recommendations or suggestions about dental care. Nevertheless it is clear that dental health in Northern Ireland is not of as high a standard as could be wished. The high proportion of edentulous persons in Northern Ireland and the lower average number of standing teeth compared with England and Wales indicate that there may be dental needs which are unmet. The regular attenders appear to be more conscious of dental health than the less regular attenders. Yet most people only visit the dentist when having trouble. It would seem there is a need for dental health education also. The planning on the provision of dental services lies outside the remit of this report. If it provides valid information about adult dental health in Northern Ireland in 1979 which can act as a basis for the future planning of dental care, it has succeeded in its appointed task.

J. R. RHODES: Department of Health and Social Services.

T. H. HAIRE: Social Research Division,
Central Economic Service,
Department of Finance.

December 1980

Characteristics of the Achieved Sample compared with the 1971 Census

ACHIEVED SAMPLE

		Number	Percentages %	Population of Northern Ireland %
SEX	Males	536	46	48
	Females	640	54	52
AGE*	16–24	184	16	20
	25–34	191	16	18
	35–44	190	16	16
	45–54	176	15	16
	55–64	181	15	14
	65–74	178	15	10
	75+	76	7	6
HEALTH AND†	Eastern	501	43	46
SOCIAL SERVICES	Western	174	15	14
BOARD	Northern	268	23	23
	Southern	233	20	17

*Percentages quoted for Northern Ireland population are based on people 16 years of age and upwards.

†Percentages quoted for Northern Ireland population are based on people 15 years of age and upwards.

Adult Dental Health Survey—Northern Ireland—1979

List of Dental Examiners

Miss K. Beamish

A. J. Casey

Mrs. E. Cooper

H. A. Dallas

W. J. Davidson

W. A. McDaid

Mrs. L. McKinney

Mrs. R. McMullin

Miss M. Madden

A. Magee

J. A. Rodgers

R. W. Tolhurst

C. A. Wilkinson

S. H. Wilson

Dental Tutors/Dental Examiners

J. R. Rhodes

Mrs. P. D. Wilson

The Dental Examination Kit

4 Plane mouth mirrors
4 Dental probes blunted to 0.7 mm*
1 Orthodontic measure
1 Chip syringe
4 Flexible Examination Lights†
2 Beakers with sealing lids
1 Sponge
1 Towel
1 Plastic Bag
1 Clinical Coat (for use on courses only)
1 Case

*As used in the 1978 Adult Dental Health Survey—UK.
†5″ Hoyt flexible dental examination light.

Area No.		Address No.		Person	

ADULT DENTAL HEALTH
NORTHERN IRELAND 1979

Introductory questionnaire

Interviewer's Name .... Inf. ....

Interviewer's No. ....

(We are interested in all people, those with all natural teeth, those with some false and those with all false teeth).

1. Could you tell me have you still got some of your natural teeth or have you lost them all?	Still has some natural teeth	4	ask (a)
	Lost them all	3	go to GREEN Q'RE
IF HAS SOME NATURAL TEETH (4)			
(a) Have you ever had any dentures, that is false teeth on a plate?	Has had dentures	4	ask (b)
	Never had dentures...............	1	go to YELLOW Q'RE
IF HAS HAD DENTURES (4)			
(b) Can I just check, have you ever had both a full upper and a full lower plate?	Both full upper and full lower	3	go to GREEN Q'RE
	Has not	2	go to PINK Q'RE

INTERVIEWER SEE OVER PAGE

2. INTERVIEW RESPONSE

Interview achieved	1 see (a)
Refusal	2
Not contact	3 see (b)
Other	4

(a) IF INTERVIEW ACHIEVED (1)

	Day	Mth
Date of interview		

(b) IF INTERVIEW NOT ACHIEVED (2, 3 or 4)
Please Give Best Estimate of Informant's Age, Sex and Dental Status

Age				Sex			Dental Status		
16–34	35–54	55+	DK	M	F	DK	Some natural teeth	No natural teeth	DK
1	2	3	4	1	2	3	1	2	3

3. DENTAL EXAMINATION RESPONSE

Informant has no natural teeth	1
Examination achieved	2 see (a)
Refusal at end of interview	3
Refusal later	4
Non contact for examination	5
Other	6

Informant has some natural teeth

(a) IF EXAMINATION ACHIEVED (2)

	Day	Mth
Date of dental examination		

Time of day for dental examination

Before 2 o'clock	1
2 o'clock but before 5 o'clock	2
5 o'clock or later	3

98

Area No.			Address No.			Person

ADULT DENTAL HEALTH
NORTHERN IRELAND 1979

Interview questionnaire 1

People with natural teeth only

Interviewer's Name .... Inf. ....

Interviewer's No. ....

I'd like to start by talking about how your teeth are at the moment.

1. Many people suffer from toothache at one time or another. During the last four weeks have you had a toothache at all or not?	Had toothache	1
	Not	2
2. During the last four weeks have you lost any fillings or have any bits broken off your teeth?	Fillings lost/tooth broken	1
	None	2
3. Do you think any of your teeth are at all loose?	Some loose	1
	None	2
4. When you are eating or drinking are there any teeth that you avoid using?	Avoids some	1 ask (a)
	Does not	2

IF AVOIDS SOME (1)

(a) What is the main reason for you avoiding those teeth?

5. (Can I just check) do you think any of your teeth are decayed at the moment?	Teeth decayed	1
	Not	2

Dental health is not only to do with teeth but with gums as well.

6. Are your gums swollen at all at the moment?	Gums swollen	1
	Not	2
7. Are your gums inflamed, that is redder than usual, at the moment?	Gums inflamed	1
	Not	2
8. During the last four weeks have your gums bled at all for example when you brushed your teeth or at any other time?	Gums bled	1
	Have not	2
9. Do you have any other sort of trouble with your gums at the moment?	Other trouble	1 ask (a)
	Not	2

IF OTHER TROUBLE (1)

(a) What other trouble do you have?

100

10. If you were to go to the dentist tomorrow do you think you would need any treatment or not?	Need treatment	1	ask (a)
	Not	2	
IF NEED TREATMENT (1)			
(a) What sort of treatment do you think you would need? PROMPT AS NEC. CODE ALL THAT APPLY	Fillings	1	
	Extractions	2	
	Fillings/extractions but DK which.	3	
	Other (SPECIFY)	4	
11(a) If you went to the dentist with an aching back tooth would you prefer the dentist to take it out or to fill it? PROMPT AS NEC. "Supposing it could be filled"	Take it out	1	
	Fill it	2	
	Other (SPECIFY)	3	
(b) If you went to the dentist with an aching front tooth would you prefer the dentist to take it out or to fill it? PROMPT AS NEC. "Supposing it could be filled"	Take it out	1	
	Fill it	2	
	Other (SPECIFY)	3	
12. You told me earlier that you've never had any dentures but when people lose some of their own teeth they may need a denture to replace them.			
(a) Do you find the thought of having a partial denture to replace **some** of your natural teeth . . . RUNNING PROMPT	. . . very upsetting	1	
	a little upsetting	2	
	or not at all upsetting	3	
(b) A lot of people eventually have their own teeth out and have full dentures. Do you find the thought of losing **all** your own teeth and having full dentures . . . RUNNING PROMPT	. . . very upsetting	1	
	a little upsetting	2	
	or not at all upsetting	3	
13. Do you think at sometime you will have to have full dentures or do you think you will always keep some of your natural teeth?	Have full dentures	1	ask (a)
	Keep natural teeth	2	
	D.K.	3	
IF HAVE FULL DENTURES (1)			
(a) At what age do you think you'll first need full dentures? PROMPT AS NECESSARY	70's or more	7	
	60's	6	
	50's	5	
	40's	4	
	30's	3	
	20's	2	

101

14. Thinking of the people you know around your age about how many of them have full dentures; would you say it was . . .

RUNNING PROMPT

. . . All or most of them	1
Some of them	2
very few or none of them	3

15. Whether or not teeth are lost is due partly to how healthy they are and different people have different ideas as to what things help to keep teeth healthy. I'd like to talk about some things people have mentioned. Can you tell me how important you consider them for keeping teeth healthy.

HAND OVER CARD A

Would you say that . . .

	FOR KEEPING TEETH HEALTHY				
	very important	fairly important	not very important	not at all important	D.K.
(i) Not eating sweets is	1	2	3	4	5
(ii) Regular visits to the dentist are	1	2	3	4	5
(iii) Cleaning teeth regularly is	1	2	3	4	5
(iv) Having fluoride in the water is	1	2	3	4	5

Now I'd like to talk a little about cleaning your teeth.

16(a) How often do you clean your teeth nowadays?

.................per...................

Never	9	go to Q.17
Once a day	1	
Twice a day	2	
More than twice a day	3	
Other (SPECIFY)	4	

(b) At what time of day do you clean them?

Before breakfast	1
After breakfast	2
Mid-day	3
Tea time	4
After evening meal	5
Last thing at night	6
Other (SPECIFY)	7

IF MORNING AND NO BREAKFAST RING 'AFTER BREAKFAST' (2)

(c) About how long ago did you start using the toothbrush you've got now? Was it . . .

RUNNING PROMPT

less than 3 months	1
3 months, but less than 6 months .	2
6 months, but less than a year	3
or a year or more ago?	4
D.K.	5
No toothbrush	6

(e) Do you use toothpaste, toothpowder or something else to clean your teeth?

Toothpaste	1	ask (f)
Toothpowder	2	
Other (SPECIFY)	3	ask (g)

102

IF TOOTHPASTE OR TOOTHPOWDER (1 or 2)

(f) Thinking of the toothpaste (toothpowder) you use at the moment does it contain fluoride or not?

Contains fluoride	1	
Does not	2	ask (g)
Don't know	3	

(g) (Can I just check) do you ever use anything else to clean your teeth such as dental floss or woodsticks?

Dental floss	1
Woodsticks	2
Other (SPECIFY)	3

Can I talk now about your childhood dental experiences.

17. When you were a child how much encouragement were you given to clean your teeth? Were you given . . .

a great deal	1
a fair amount	2
not much	3
or no encouragement at all?	4

18. When you were a child (that is before you were 16) did you ever go to a dentist?

Went to a dentist	1	ask (a)
Did not	2	go to Q.19

IF WENT TO A DENTIST (1)

(a) Did you go to the school dentist, to some other dentist or both?

School dentist	1	ask (c)
Other dentist	2	ask (b)
Both	3	

IF WENT TO OTHER DENTIST OR BOTH (2), (3)

(b) (Excluding visits to the school dentist) as a child, did you go to the dentist for

a regular check up	1	
an occasional check up	2	ask (c)
or only when you were having trouble with you teeth?	3	
Other (SPECIFY)	4	

(c) Thinking now about any treatment you had then. Did you have any teeth filled before you were 16?

Teeth filled	1
Not	2
D.K./can't remember	3

(d) Did you have any teeth taken out when you were that age?

Teeth taken out	1
Not	2
D.K./can't remember	3

(e) Nowadays children sometimes have a brace fitted or teeth taken out to help straighten their teeth. Did you have any treatment to straighten or improve the appearance of your teeth?

Had treatment	1	ask (f)
Did not	2	
D.K./can't remember	3	

IF HAD TREATMENT (1)

(f) Did you have a brace fitted, teeth taken out, both of these or some other treatment?

Brace fitted	1
Teeth taken out	2
Both	3
Other (SPECIFY)	4

103

We've talked a little about childhood and now I'd like to talk about the dental experiences you've had through the whole of your life.

IF TEETH FILLED WHEN CHILD (Q.18(c) CODE (1)) RING (1) AND ASK (a–b)

19. Have you ever had any teeth filled?	Teeth filled	1	ask (a–b)
	Not	2	Go to Q.20

IF TEETH FILLED (1)

(a) Have you ever had an injection in your gum to kill the pain of a filling?	Injection in gum.................	1	
	Not	2	

(b) Have you ever had an injection in your arm to kill the pain of a filling?	Injection in arm	1	ask (c)
	Not	2	see (c)

IF HAD INJECTION (a) OR (b) CODE (1)

(c) Do you usually have an injection when you're having a filling done?	Usually	1	
	Not	2	

IF TEETH TAKEN OUT WHEN CHILD (Q.18 (d) CODE (1)) RING (1) AND ASK (a–c)

20. Have you ever had any teeth taken out?	Teeth taken out	1	ask (a–c)
	Not	2	Go to Q.21

IF TEETH TAKEN OUT (1)

(a) Have you ever had gas to have teeth taken out?	Had gas	1	
	Not	2	

(b) Have you ever had an injection in your gum to have teeth taken out?	Injection in gum.................	1	
	Not	2	

(c) Have you ever had an injection in your arm to have teeth taken out?	Injection in arm	1	
	Not	2	

21. Have you ever had an X-ray taken of your teeth?	Had X-ray	1	ask (a)
	Not	2	

IF HAD X-RAY (1)

(a) Do you usually have an X-ray taken of your teeth when you go to the dentist?	Usually has X-ray	1	
	Does not	2	

22. The wisdom teeth, which are the very back teeth, often come through later than the other teeth and sometimes don't come through at all. Can you tell me which of your wisdom teeth have, at sometime, come through.

Has the one at the . . . come through or not?		top left	top right	bottom left	bottom right	
	Come through	1	1	1	1	ask (a)
	Not come through..	2	2	2	2	
	D.K.	3	3	3	3	
IF COME THROUGH (1)						
(a) Have you still got the . . . widom tooth or have you had it out since?	still got it	4	4	4	4	
	taken out	5	5	5	5	

As well as treating people's teeth dentists can give advice to their patients on caring for their teeth and mouths and on preventing disease.

23. Has a dentist or any of his staff demonstrated to you the best way to clean your teeth?	Demonstrated	1	ask (a)
	Not	2	
IF DEMONSTRATED (1)			
(a) Who was it who demonstrated teeth cleaning to you? Was it . . .	a dentist	1	
	a dental nurse or hygienist	2	
RUNNING PROMPT	or somebody else (SPECIFY)	3	
24. Has a dentist or any of his staff ever given you any advice on caring for your gums?	Given advice	1	ask (a–b)
	Not	2	
IF GIVEN ADVICE (1)			
(a) Who was it who gave you the advice? Was it . . .	a dentist	1	
	a dental nurse or hygienist	2	
	or somebody else (SPECIFY)	3	
(b) What advice did he/she give you?			
25. Has a dentist or any of his staff ever advised you about eating sweets or other sugary things?	Advised	1	ask (a–b)
	Not	2	
IF ADVISED (1)			
(a) Who was it who gave you the advice? Was it . . .	a dentist	1	
	a dental nurse or hygienist	2	
	or somebody else (SPECIFY)	3	
(b) What did he/she say?			

Another part of dentist's work is to provide treatment to improve the appearance of teeth which are crooked or protruding.

SHOW CARD A

26(a) How important do you think it is that children with crooked or protruding teeth should have them straightened. Do you think it is . . .	very important	1
	fairly important	2
RUNNING PROMPT	not very important	3
	or not at all important?	4

(b) How important do you think it is that adults with crooked or protruding teeth should have them straightened. Do you think it is . . .
RUNNING PROMPT

very important 1
fairly important 2
not very important 3
or not at all important? 4

— see (c)

IF ONE LESS IMPORTANT THAN OTHER
(c) Why do you think it is less important for . . . to have their teeth straightened?

27. How do you feel about your own teeth; are you satisfied or not satisfied with the way they look?

Satisfied 1   go to Q.28
Not satisfied 2   ask (a–b)

IF NOT SATISFIED (2)
(a) What is it about the way your teeth look that you're not satisfied with?

(b) Have you ever talked to a dentist about the appearance of your teeth?

Talked to dentist 1   ask (c)
Not 2   ask (d)

IF TALKED TO DENTIST (1)
(c) What did the dentist say?

IF NOT (2)
(d) Is there any reason why you haven't talked to a dentist about the appearance of your teeth?

I'd like to talk now about going to the dentist.

28. Have you been to the dentist since the beginning of February, that's about six months ago?

Yes 1   ask (a)
No 2   ask (b)

IF YES (1)
(a) (Can I just check) are you in the middle of a course of treatment now or not?

In middle of treatment 1
Not 2

— go to Q.29

IF NO (2)
(b) Have you been to the dentist since last September, that'a about a year ago?

Yes 1   go to Q.29
No 2   ask (c)

106

IF NO (b) CODE (2)

(c) About how long ago was your last visit to the dentist?

More than 1 up to 2 years ago ...	1	ask (d)
More than 2 up to 3 years ago ...	2	
More than 3 up to 5 years ago ...	3	go to Q.29
More than that (SPECIFY)	4	
Never	5	go to Q.150

PROMPT IF NEC.

....

IF Q.28(c) CODE (1)

(d) Was this before or after 1 September 1978

Before April 1st	1
April 1st or after	2

29. The last time you went to the dentist what made you go? Was it because you were having some trouble with your teeth or for a check up or for some other reason?

Trouble with teeth	1	ask (a)
Check up	2	
Other (SPECIFY)	3	

IF TROUBLE WITH TEETH (1)

(a) Did you have toothache or did you have some other trouble with your teeth?

Toothache	1
Other (SPECIFY)	2

30. When people go to the dentist for a check up or because they've got trouble with their teeth, they sometimes have to make more than one visit for the dentist to carry out any treatment they might need.

When you last went to the dentist how many visits did you have to make?

One visit	1
Two visits	2
Three visits	3
Four visits	4
Five or more..................	5

31. (Can I just check) during the visit(s) you made to the dentist for that course of treatment did you have any . . .

	Yes	No	D.K.
X-rays taken...................	1	2	3
Teeth filled	1	2	3
Teeth taken out	1	2	3
Teeth scaled (scraped, cleaned) and polished	1	2	3
Other treatment (SPECIFY)	1	2	3

INDIVIDUAL PROMPT

32. Was your treatment under the Health Service, was it private or was it something else?

National Health Service	1	
Private	2	ask (b)
N.H.S. and private	3	ask (a–b)
Community Dental Service	4	
Armed Forces..................	5	
Other (SPECIFY)	6	

107

IF N.H.S. AND PRIVATE (3)
(a) What treatment did you have privately?

IF ANY PRIVATE (2 or 3)
(b) What was the main reason for you having this treatment done privately?

SEE EXTRA QUESTION—N.I. QUESTIONS

33. How much did the treatment cost you?	Cost (SPECIFY)	1	ask (a)
	Nothing	2	ask (b)
....	D.K.	3	go to Q.34

IF PAID FOR TREATMENT (1)
(a) Did the treatment cost more than you expected, about what you expected or less than you expected?

More than expected	1	
About what expected	2	go to Q.34
Less than expected	3	
Other (SPECIFY)	4	

IF NOTHING (2)
(b) Why didn't it cost you anything?

PROMPT AS NEC.

No treatment	1	go to Q.34
Under 21, pregnant or nursing mother	2	ask (c)
Other (SPECIFY)	3	

(c) When you went to the dentist did you expect the treatment would be free?

Yes	1
No	2

34. Thinking about the dental practice you went to for your last treatment, was that the first time you had been to that dentist or group of dentists or had you been there before?	First time	1	ask (c)
	Been before	2	ask (a–b)

IF BEEN BEFORE (2)
(a) For about how many years have you been going to that dentist or group of dentists?

Less than a year	1
One year less than two	2
Two years less than five	3
Five years or more	4
D.K./Can't remember	5

(b) Does the dentist send you a reminder when it is time to go for your next check up?

Sends reminder	1	go to Q.35
Does not	2	ask (c)

IF DOES NOT SEND REMINDER (2) OR FIRST TIME (1)

(c) When you make an appointment to see the dentist do you usually make it . . .

. . . at the end of your previous treatment	1	go to Q.35
some time before the date that you want the appointment	2	ask (d)
or when you want to see the dentist as soon as possible	3	
Other (SPECIFY)	4	go to Q.35

IF CODE (2) OR (3)

(d) Last time you wanted to see the dentist about how long did you have to wait for an appointment?

35. How did you come to choose that particular dentist?

Can't remember 9

USE PROMPTS

36. In the last five years have you had any difficulty getting any treatment under the Health Service?

Had difficulty	1	ask (a–b)
Not	2	
Not tried	3	

IF HAD DIFFICULTY (1)

(a) What treatment couldn't you get?
ALL OF IT/
PART OF IT
IF PART, WHAT PART?

(b) What did you do about it?

37. In general do you go to the dentist for . . .

a regular check up	1	go to Q.38
an occasional check up	2	
or only when you're having trouble with your teeth	3	

IF DOES NOT GO FOR A REGULAR CHECK UP (2 or 3)

(a) What is the main reason for you not going for a regular check up?

(b) (You've told me the main reason for you not going for a regular check up) now I'd like to ask about the kinds of circumstances when you would go to the dentist. Would you go to the dentist if you had . . .

	YES	NO
Occasional twinges of toothache	1	2
A tooth which felt loose	1	2
Not been to the dentist for a long time	1	2
INDIVIDUAL PROMPT A swollen face	1	2
Sore gums	1	2
Toothache which kept you awake at night . . .	1	2
A gumboil	1	2
A tooth with a piece broken off	1	2
Gums which bled occasionally	1	2

38. Would you say that nowadays you go to the dentist more often, about the same or less often than you did five years ago?	More often	1	ask (a)
	About the same	2	
	Less often	3	ask (a)

IF MORE OR LESS OFTEN (1 or 3)
(a) What has made you go more (less) often?

I'd like to talk generally now about the cost of dental treatment under the Health Service.

39. When you go to the dentist to have treatment do you normally have some idea of how much it's going to cost you?	Has some idea	1
	Does not	2

40. Do you know where you can find out about Health Service dental charges?	Yes	1	ask (a)
	No	2	
IF YES (1) (a) Where can you find out?	Dentist	1	
	G.P.O.	2	
	Other (SPECIFY)	3	

41. When you have to pay at the dentist does he usually tell you what the total cost is made up of?	Yes	1
	No	2
	Never paid	3

110

42. I'd like you to look at these different treatments and tell me how much you think each would cost, whether it would cost nothing or whether it would cost £2 or less, between £2 and £5, or £5 or more?

SHOW CARDS B AND C	TREATMENT WOULD COST				
COURSE OF TREATMENT (B)	Nothing (Free)	£2 or less	Between £2 and £5	£5 or more	D.K.
Exam, 2 teeth out	1	2	3	4	5
Exam, 1 large filling, 1 tooth out...............	1	2	3	4	5
Examination only	1	2	3	4	5
Exam, 2 X-rays, scale and polish, 1 small filling ..	1	2	3	4	5
Exam, 4 teeth out, new dentures fitted	1	2	3	4	5
Exam, 2 X-rays, 6 teeth out, gas	1	2	3	4	5
Repair of cracked denture	1	2	3	4	5
Exam, 2 X-rays, scale and polish	1	2	3	4	5

43. For most kinds of treatment under the Health Service the patient pays the full cost up to the first £7.

(a) As a maximum charge do you think £7 is: too high 1

    RUNNING PROMPT   about right 2

    or too low? 3

(b) A few kinds of dental treatment are rather expensive and so the patient has to pay more than £7 to be treated under the Health Service.

Do you know what kinds of treatment   Yes 1   ask (c)
cost the patient more than £7?

    No 2

IF YES (1)
(c) What kinds of treatment cost the patient more than £7?

44. Some people get exemption from dental charges   Yes 1   ask (a)
so that all the treatment they have is free.
Do you know what kinds of people get free   No 2
treatment?

IF YES (1)
(a) What kinds of people get free treatment?   Pregnant or nursing mothers...... 1

    Other (SPECIFY) 2

111

45. People have mentioned all sorts of things that make them put off going to the dentist. Can you look at this card and tell me for each of the statements I read out whether these things apply to you very much, a fair amount, not very much or not at all.

SHOW CARD D I put off going to the dentist because . . .	APPLIES TO ME				
	very much	a fair amount	not very much	not at all	D.K.
I'm scared of the dentist	1	2	3	4	5
It's difficult to get time off work	1	2	3	4	5
I don't like having fillings	1	2	3	4	5
It's too expensive to go too often	1	2	3	4	5
I haven't got a regular dentist	1	2	3	4	5
I can't be bothered really	1	2	3	4	5
Of the thought of having teeth out	1	2	3	4	5
It's difficult to get an appointment...........	1	2	3	4	5
It's a long way to go	1	2	3	4	5

46. What do you find most unpleasant about going to the dentist?

GO TO N.I. QUESTIONS

47. Are there any other comments you would like to make about your teeth or going to the dentist?

CLASSIFICATION — TO ALL

		Day	Month	Year

150. (a) Date of birth of informant

(b) Sex of informant

	Year
Male	1
Female	2

(c) Age informant finished full time education

14 years or less	4
15 years	5
16 years	6
17 years	7
18 years or more	8
Still in f/t education	9

(d) Employment status of informant

Full time	1
Part time	2
Not in employment	3

(e) Marital status of informant

Married	1
Single	2
W/S/D.......................	3

(f) What is the occupation of the informant?
(GIVE OCCUPATION AND INDUSTRY)

(g) IS THE INFORMANT HOH OR NOT?

Informant HOH	1	go to Q.152
Not	2	go to Q.151

151. What is the occupation of the HOH?
(GIVE OCCUPATION AND INDUSTRY)

152. (a) Grateful for their help—asking for a little more in order to complete the picture.

(b) Some things only a dentist looking at your teeth would see.

(c) Asking anybody who has some teeth if dentist can come back in a few days time.

(d) He won't comment on your teeth at all, to you or anyone else (ethics).

(e) Result will help to estimate the need for treatment.

(f) Reassurance that it will not hurt at all, and interviewer will be there.

(g) Length of time for examination.

Willing to have examination . . . . . . | 1 | see (h)

Not . . . . | 2 | see (j)

IF WILLING (1)
(h) appointment details

GIVE INFORMANT APPOINTMENT CARD

IF NOT WILLING (2)
(j) NOTE COMMENTS

	Area No.		Address No.		Person

ADULT DENTAL HEALTH
NORTHERN IRELAND 1979

Interview questionnaire 2

Has (Had) partial dentures

Interviewer's Name .... Inf. ....

Interviewer's No. ....

I'd like to talk first about your natural teeth and how they are at the moment.

1.	Many people suffer from toothache at one time or another. During the last four weeks have you had a toothache at all or not?	00 Had toothache	1
		Not	2
2.	During the last four weeks have you lost any fillings or have any bits broken off your teeth?	Fillings lost/tooth broken	1
		None	2
3.	Do you think any of your teeth are at all loose?	Some loose	1
		None	2
4.	When you are eating or drinking are there any teeth that you avoid using?	Avoids some	1 ask (a)
		Does not	2

IF AVOIDS SOME (1)
(a) What is the main reason for you avoiding those teeth?

5.	(Can I just check) do you think any of your teeth are decayed at the moment?	Teeth decayed	1
		Not	2

Dental health is not only to do with teeth but with gums as well.

6.	Are your gums swollen at all at the moment?	Gums swollen	1
		Not	2
7.	Are your gums inflamed, that is redder than usual, at the moment?	Gums inflamed	1
		Not	2
8.	During the last four weeks have your gums bled at all for example when you brushed your teeth or at any other time?	Gums bled	1
		Have not	2
9.	Do you have any other sort of trouble with your gums at the moment?	Other trouble	1 ask (a)
		Not	2

IF OTHER TROUBLE (1)
(a) What other trouble do you have?

10. If you were to go to the dentist tomorrow do you think you would need any treatment or not?	Need treatment	1	ask (a)
	Not	2	
IF NEED TREATMENT (1)			
(a) What sort of treatment do you think you would need? PROMPT AS NEC. CODE ALL THAT APPLY	Fillings	1	
	Extractions	2	
	Fillings/extractions but DK which.	3	
	Other (SPECIFY)	4	

11(a) If you went to the dentist with an aching back tooth would you prefer the dentist to take it out or to fill it? PROMPT AS NEC. "Supposing it could be filled"	Take it out	1
	Fill it	2
	Other (SPECIFY)	3
(b) If you went to the dentist with an aching front tooth would you prefer the dentist to take it out or to fill it? PROMPT AS NEC. "Supposing it could be filled"	Take it out	1
	Fill it	2
	Other (SPECIFY)	3

12(a)	DNA	
(b) A lot of people eventually have their own teeth out and have full dentures. Do you find the thought of losing **all** your own teeth and having full dentures ... RUNNING PROMPT	... very upsetting	1
	a little upsetting	2
	or not at all upsetting	3

13. Do you think at sometime you will have to have full dentures or do you think you will always keep some of your natural teeth?	Have full dentures	1	ask (a)
	Keep natural teeth	2	
	D.K.	3	
IF HAVE FULL DENTURES (1)			
(a) At what age do you think you'll first need full dentures?	70's or more	7	
	60's	6	
PROMPT AS NECESSARY	50's	5	
	40's	4	
	30's	3	
	20's	2	

14. Thinking of the people you know around your age about how many of them have full dentures; would you say it was ...	... All or most of them	1
	Some of them...................	2
RUNNING PROMPT	very few or none of them	3

117

15. Whether or not teeth are lost is due partly to how healthy they are and different people have different ideas as to what things help to keep teeth healthy.
I'd like to talk about some things people have mentioned. Can you tell me how important you consider them for keeping natural teeth healthy.

HAND OVER CARD A Would you say that . . .	FOR KEEPING NATURAL TEETH HEALTHY				
	very important	fairly important	not very important	not at all important	D.K.
(i) Not eating sweets is	1	2	3	4	5
(ii) Regular visits to the dentist are	1	2	3	4	5
(iii) Cleaning teeth regularly is	1	2	3	4	5
(iv) Having fluoride in the water is	1	2	3	4	5

Now I'd like to talk a little about cleaning your natural teeth.

16(a) How often do you clean your teeth nowadays?

Never	9	go to Q.17
Once a day	1	
Twice a day	2	
More than twice a day	3	
..................per.................. Other (SPECIFY)	4	

(b) At what time of day do you clean them?

Before breakfast	1
After breakfast	2
Mid-day	3
Tea time.......................	4
After evening meal	5
Last thing at night	6
Other (SPECIFY)	7

IF MORNING AND NO BREAKFAST RING 'AFTER BREAKFAST' (2)

(c) About how long ago did you start using the toothbrush you've got now? Was it . . .

less than 3 months	1
3 months, but less than 6 months	2
6 months, but less than a year....	3

RUNNING PROMPT

or a year or more ago?	4
D.K.	5
No toothbrush	6

(e) Do you use toothpaste, toothpowder or something else to clean your teeth?

Toothpaste.....................	1	ask (f)
Toothpowder...................	2	
Other (SPECIFY)	3	ask (g)

IF TOOTHPASTE OR TOOTHPOWDER (1 or 2)

(f) Thinking of the toothpaste (toothpowder) you use at the moment does it contain fluoride or not?	Contains fluoride	1	
	Does not	2	ask (g)
	Don't know	3	

(g) (Can I just check) do you ever use anything else to clean your natural teeth such as dental floss or woodsticks?	Dental floss	1	
	Woodsticks	2	
	Other (SPECIFY)	3	

Can I talk now about your childhood dental experiences.

17. When you were a child how much encouragement were you given to clean your teeth? Were you given . . .	a great deal	1	
	a fair amount	2	
	not much	3	
	or no encouragement at all?	4	

18. When you were a child (that is before you were 16) did you ever go to a dentist?	Went to a dentist...............	1	ask (a)
	Did not	2	go to Q.19

IF WENT TO A DENTIST (1)			
(a) Did you go to the school dentist, to some other dentist or both?	School dentist	1	ask (c)
	Other dentist	2	
	Both	3	ask (b)

IF WENT TO OTHER DENTIST OR BOTH (2), (3)			
(b) (Excluding visits to the school dentist) as a child, did you go to the dentist for	a regular check up..............	1	
	an occasional check up...........	2	
	or only when you were having trouble with you teeth?...........	3	ask (c)
	Other (SPECIFY)	4	

(c) Thinking now about any treatment you had then. Did you have any teeth filled before you were 16?	Teeth filled	1	
	Not	2	
	D.K./can't remember	3	

(d) Did you have any teeth taken out when you were that age?	Teeth taken out	1	
	Not	2	
	D.K./can't remember	3	

(e) Nowadays children sometimes have a brace fitted or teeth taken out to help straighten their teeth. Did you have any treatment to straighten or improve the appearance of your teeth?	Had treatment	1	ask (f)
	Did not	2	
	D.K./can't remember	3	

119

(f) Did you have a brace fitted, teeth taken out, both of these or some other treatment?

Brace fitted	1
Teeth taken out	2
Both	3
Other (SPECIFY)	4

We've talked a little about childhood and now I'd like to talk about the dental experiences you've had through the whole of your life.
IF TEETH FILLED WHEN CHILD (Q.18(c) CODE (1)) RING (1) AND ASK (a–b)

19. Have you ever had any teeth filled?

Teeth filled	1	ask (a–b)
Not	2	Go to Q.20

IF TEETH FILLED (1)
(a) Have you ever had an injection in your gum to kill the pain of a filling?

Injection in gum.................	1
Not	2

(b) Have you ever had an injection in your arm to kill the pain of a filling?

Injection in arm	1	ask (c)
Not	2	see (c)

IF HAD INJECTION (a) OR (b) CODE (1)
(c) Do you usually have an injection when you're having a filling done?

Usually	1
Not	2

IF TEETH TAKEN OUT WHEN CHILD (Q.18 (d) CODE (1)) RING (1) AND ASK (a–c)

20. Have you ever had any teeth taken out?

Teeth taken out	1	ask (a–c)
Not	2	Go to Q.21

IF TEETH TAKEN OUT (1)
(a) Have you ever had gas to have teeth taken out?

Had gas	1
Not	2

(b) Have you ever had an injection in your gum to have teeth taken out?

Injection in gum.................	1
Not	2

(c) Have you ever had an injection in your arm to have teeth taken out?

Injection in arm	1
Not	2

21. Have you ever had an X-ray taken of your teeth?

Had X-ray	1	ask (a)
Not	2	

IF HAD X-RAY (1)
(a) Do you usually have an X-ray taken of your teeth when you go to the dentist?

Usually has X-ray	1
Does not	2

22. The wisdom teeth, which are the very back teeth, often come through later than the other teeth and sometimes don't come through at all. Can you tell me which of your wisdom teeth have, at sometime, come through.

Has the one at the . . . come through or not?		top left	top right	bottom left	bottom right	
	Come through	1	1	1	1	ask (a)
	Not come through..	2	2	2	2	
	D.K.	3	3	3	3	
IF COME THROUGH (1) (a) Have you still got the . . . widom tooth or have you had it out since?	still got it	4	4	4	4	
	taken out	5	5	5	5	

As well as treating people's teeth dentists can give advice to their patients on caring for their teeth and mouths and on preventing disease.

23. Has a dentist or any of his staff demonstrated to you the best way to clean your teeth?

Demonstrated 1   ask (a)

Not 2

IF DEMONSTRATED (1)
(a) Who was it who demonstrated teeth cleaning to you? Was it . . .

RUNNING PROMPT

a dentist 1

a dental nurse or hygienist 2

or somebody else (SPECIFY) 3

24. Has a dentist or any of his staff ever given you any advice on caring for your gums?

Given advice 1   ask (a–b)

Not 2

IF GIVEN ADVICE (1)
(a) Who was it who gave you the advice? Was it . . .

RUNNING PROMPT

a dentist 1

a dental nurse or hygienist 2

or somebody else (SPECIFY) 3

(b) What advice did he/she give you?

25. Has a dentist or any of his staff ever advised you about eating sweets or other sugary things?

Advised 1   ask (a–b)

Not 2

IF ADVISED (1)
(a) Who was it who gave you the advice? Was it . . .

RUNNING PROMPT

a dentist 1

a dental nurse or hygienist 2

or somebody else (SPECIFY) 3

(b) What did he/she say?

121

Another part of dentist's work is to provide treatment to improve the appearance of teeth which are crooked or protruding.

SHOW CARD A

26(a) How important do you think it is that children with crooked or protruding teeth should have them straightened. Do you think it is . . .

RUNNING PROMPT

very important	1
fairly important	2
not very important	3
or not at all important?	4

(b) How important do you think it is that adults with crooked or protruding teeth should have them straightened. Do you think it is . . .

RUNNING PROMPT

very important	1
fairly important	2
not very important	3
or not at all important?	4

see (c)

IF ONE LESS IMPORTANT THAN OTHER

(c) Why do you think it is less important for . . . to have their teeth straightened?

27. How do you feel about your own teeth; are you satisfied or not satisfied with the way they look?

Satisfied	1	go to Q.28
Not satisfied	2	ask (a–b)
Informant says DNA	3	go to Q.28

IF NOT SATISFIED (2)

(a) What is it about the ay your teeth look that you're not satisfied with?

(b) Have you ever talked to a dentist about the appearance of your teeth?

Talked to dentist	1	ask (c)
Not	2	ask (d)

IF TALKED TO DENTIST (1)

(c) What did the dentist say?

IF NOT (2)

(d) Is there any reason why you haven't talked to a dentist about the appearance of your teeth?

I'd like to talk now about going to the dentist.

28. Have you been to the dentist since the beginning of February, that's about six months ago?

Yes .... 1 ask (a)

No .... 2 ask (b)

IF YES (1)
(a) (Can I just check) are you in the middle of a course of treatment now or not?

In middle of treatment 1

Not 2

go to Q.29

IF NO (2)
(b) Have you been to the dentist since last September, that'a about a year ago?

Yes .... 1 go to Q.29

No .... 2 ask (c)

IF NO (b) CODE (2)
(c) About how long ago was your last visit to the dentist?

More than 1 up to 2 years ago ... 1 ask (d)

More than 2 up to 3 years ago ... 2

PROMPT IF NEC.

More than 3 up to 5 years ago ... 3

go to Q.29

More than that (SPECIFY) 4

Never .... 5 go to Q.150

IF Q.28(c) CODE (1)
(d) Was this before or after 1 September 1978

Before April 1st 1

April 1st or after 2

29. The last time you went to the dentist what made you go? Was it because you were having some trouble with your teeth or for a check up or for some other reason?

Trouble with teeth .... 1 ask (a)

Check up 2

Other (SPECIFY) 3

IF TROUBLE WITH TEETH (1)
(a) Did you have toothache or did you have some other trouble with your teeth?

Toothache 1

Other (SPECIFY) 2

30. When people go to the dentist for a check up or because they've got trouble with their teeth, they sometimes have to make more than one visit for the dentist to carry out any treatment they might need.

When you last went to the dentist how many visits did you have to make?

One visit 1

Two visits 2

Three visits 3

Four visits 4

Five or more................... 5

31. (Can I just check) during the visit(s) you made to the dentist for that course of treatment did you have any . . .	YES	NO	D.K.
X-rays taken......................	1	2	3
Teeth filled	1	2	3
INDIVIDUAL PROMPT Teeth taken out	1	2	3
Teeth scaled (scraped, cleaned) and polished	1	2	3
New dentures fitted............................	1	2	3
Old dentures repaired	1	2	3
Other treatment (SPECIFY)	1	2	3

32. Was your treatment under the Health Service, was it private or was it something else?

National Health Service	1	
Private	2	ask (b)
N.H.S. and private	3	ask (a–b)
Community Dental Service	4	
Armed Forces	5	
Other (SPECIFY)	6	

IF N.H.S. AND PRIVATE (3)
(a) What treatment did you have privately?

IF ANY PRIVATE (2 or 3)
(b) What was the main reason for you having this treatment done privately?

SEE EXTRA QUESTION—N.I. QUESTIONS

33. How much did the treatment cost you?

Cost (SPECIFY)	1	ask (a)
Nothing	2	ask (b)
D.K.	3	go to Q.34

IF PAID FOR TREATMENT (1)
(a) Did the treatment cost more than you expected, about what you expected or less than you expected?

More than expected	1	
About what expected	2	go to Q.34
Less than expected	3	
Other (SPECIFY)	4	

IF NOTHING (2)
(b) Why didn't it cost you anything?

No treatment.....................	1	go to Q.34
Under 21, pregnant or nursing mother	2	
Other (SPECIFY)	3	ask (c)

(c) When you went to the dentist did you expect the treatment would be free?

Yes	1
No	2

124

34. Thinking about the dental practice you went to for your last treatment, was that the first time you had been to that dentist or group of dentists or had you been there before?

First time 1   ask (c)

Been before 2   ask (a–b)

IF BEEN BEFORE (2)

(a) For about how many years have you been going to that dentist or group of dentists?

Less than a year 1

One year less than two 2

Two years less than five 3

Five years or more 4

D.K./Can't remember 5

(b) Does the dentist send you a reminder when it is time to go for your next check up?

Sends reminder 1   go to Q.35

Does not 2   ask (c)

IF DOES NOT SEND REMINDER (2) OR FIRST TIME (1)

(c) When you make an appointment to see the dentist do you usually make it . . .

. . . at the end of your previous treatment 1   go to Q.35

some time before the date that you want the appointment 2

or when you want to see the dentist as soon as possible 3   ask (d)

Other (SPECIFY) 4   go to Q.35

IF CODE (2) OR (3)

(d) Last time you wanted to see the dentist about how long did you have to wait for an appointment?

35. How did you come to choose that particular dentist?

Can't remember 9

USE PROMPTS

36. In the last five years have you had any difficulty getting any treatment under the Health Service?

Had difficulty 1   ask (a–b)

Not 2

Not tried 3

IF HAD DIFFICULTY (1)

(a) What treatment couldn't you get?
    ALL OF IT/
    PART OF IT
    IF PART, WHAT PART?

(b) What did you do about it?

37. In general do you go to the dentist for . . .

a regular check up	. . . .	1	go to Q.38
an occasional check up	. . . .	2	
or only when you're having trouble with your teeth	. . . .	3	

IF DOES NOT GO FOR A REGULAR CHECK UP (2 or 3)

(a) What is the main reason for you not going for a regular check up?

(b) (You've told me the main reason for you not going for a regular check up) now I'd like to ask about the kinds of circumstances when you would go to the dentist. Would you go to the dentist if you had . . .

	YES	NO
Occasional twinges of toothache	1	2
A tooth which felt loose	1	2
Not been to the dentist for a long time	1	2
A swollen face	1	2
Sore gums	1	2
Toothache which kept you awake at night . . .	1	2
A gumboil	1	2
A tooth with a piece broken off	1	2
Gums which bled occasionally	1	2

38. Would you say that nowadays you go to the dentist more often, about the same or less often than you did five years ago?

More often	. . . .	1	ask (a)
About the same	. . . .	2	
Less often	. . . .	3	ask (a)

IF MORE OR LESS OFTEN (1 or 3)

(a) What has made you go more (less) often?

I'd like to talk generally now about the cost of dental treatment under the Health Service.

39. When you go to the dentist to have treatment do you normally have some idea of how much it's going to cost you?

Has some idea	. . . .	1
Does not	. . . .	2

40. Do you know where you can find out about Health Service dental charges?

Yes	. . . .	1	ask (a)
No	. . . .	2	

IF YES (1)

(a) Where can you find out?

Dentist	. . . .	1
G.P.O.	. . . .	2
Other (SPECIFY)	. . . .	3

41. When you have to pay at the dentist does he usually tell you what the total cost is made up of?

Yes	1
No	2
Never paid	3

42. I'd like you to look at these different treatments and tell me how much you think each would cost, whether it would cost nothing or whether it would cost £2 or less, between £2 and £5, or £5 or more?

SHOW CARDS B AND C

COURSE OF TREATMENT (B)

	TREATMENT WOULD COST				
	Nothing (Free)	£2 or less	Between £2 and £5	£5 or more	D.K.
Exam, 2 teeth out	1	2	3	4	5
Exam, 1 large filling, 1 tooth out...............	1	2	3	4	5
Examination only	1	2	3	4	5
Exam, 2 X-rays, scale and polish, 1 sall filling	1	2	3	4	5
Exam, 4 teeth out, new dentures fitted	1	2	3	4	5
Exam, 2 X-rays, 6 teeth out, gas	1	2	3	4	5
Repair of cracked denture	1	2	3	4	5
Exam, 2 X-rays, scale and polish	1	2	3	4	5

43. For most kinds of treatment under the Health Service the patient pays the full cost up to the first £7.

(a) As a maximum charge do you think £7 is:

RUNNING PROMPT

too high	1
about right	2
or too low?	3

(b) A few kinds of dental treatment are rather expensive and so the patient has to pay more than £7 to be treated under the Health Service.

Do you know what kinds of treatment cost the patient more than £7?

Yes	1	ask (c)
No	2	

IF YES (1)
(c) What kinds of treatment cost the patient more than £7?

44. Some people get exemption from dental charges so that all the treatment they have is free. Do you know what kinds of people get free treatment?

Yes	1	ask (a)
No	2	

IF YES (1)
(a) What kinds of people get free treatment?

Pregnant or nursing mothers......	1
Other (SPECIFY)	2

127

45. People have mentioned all sorts of things that make them put off going to the dentist. Can you look at this card and tell me for each of the statements I read out whether these things apply to you very much, a fair amount, not very much or not at all.

SHOW CARD D	APPLIES TO ME				
I put off going to the dentist because . . .	very much	a fair amount	not very much	not at all	D.K.
I'm scared of the dentist	1	2	3	4	5
It's difficult to get time off work	1	2	3	4	5
I don't like having fillings	1	2	3	4	5
It's too expensive to go too often	1	2	3	4	5
I haven't got a regular dentist	1	2	3	4	5
I can't be bothered really	1	2	3	4	5
Of the thought of having teeth out	1	2	3	4	5
It's difficult to get an appointment	1	2	3	4	5
It's a long way to go	1	2	3	4	5

46. What do you find most unpleasant about going to the dentist?

GO TO N.I. QUESTIONS

47.

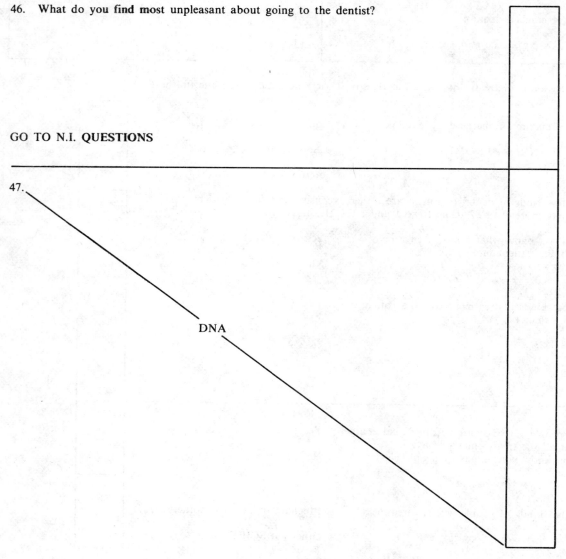

DNA

128

I would like to talk now about your partial dentures (false teeth).

50(a) Have you ever had a top plate?	Has (had) top plate.............	1	
	Not	2	
(b) Have you ever had a bottom plate?	Has (had) bottom plate	1	
	Not	2	

ASK FOR EACH PLATE AS APPROPRIATE

		Top Plate	Bottom Plate	
(c) Is the top plate (bottom plate) a full plate or not?	Full plate	1	1	
	Not	2	2	ask (d)
IF NOT (2) (d) Has the top plate (bottom plate) got some front teeth on it, or is it all back teeth?	Some front	1	1	
	All back	2	2	

51.   DNA

People with fulldentures sometimes get on better with one plate than the other so I'd like to talk about your top and bottom plates separately.

		Top Plate	Bottom Plate	
52. Have you worn your top plate (bottom plate) at all during the last four weeks?	Yes, worn	1	1	ask (a–c)
	Not	2*	2*	
IF WORN IN LAST FOUR WEEKS (1) (a) (Sometimes people don't get on very well with a new denture and go back to wearing their old one): Is the top plate (bottom plate) that you wear now the most recent one you've had or not?	Wears most recent	8	8	
	Wears old one	9	9	
(I'd like to talk about the denture you wear) (b) Do you usually keep your top plate (bottom plate) in at night?	In at night	3	3	
	Not	4	4	
(c) Do you wear your top plate (bottom plate) from the time you get up to when you go to bed?	All daytime	5	5	
	Not	6*	6*	

INTERVIEWER

    FOR PLATES NOT WORN IN LAST FOUR WEEKS (2) ASK Q'S 53–54.

    FOR PLATES NOT WORN ALL DAYTIME (6) ASK Q'S 55–56.

    FOR PLATES WORN ALL DAYTIME (5) ASK Q'S 57–62.

FOR PLATES NOT WORN IN LAST FOUR WEEKS Q.52 CODE (2)

		Top Plate	Bottom Plate	
53. Have you still got your top plate (bottom plate)?	Still got	1	1	ask (a)
	Not	2	2	ask (b)
IF STILL GOT (1) (a) Why don't you wear your top plate (bottom plate)?	Denture replaced with fixed appliance ..	1	1	go to Q.150
IF NOT (2) (b) What happened to your top plate (bottom plate)?	Denture replaced with fixed appliance ..	1	1	go to Q.150
54. Have you ever had a top plate (bottom plate) that you could wear?	Had plate............	1	1	Check other plate. Go to Q.63 for this plate.
	Not	2	2	

FOR PLATES NOT WORN ALL DAYTIME Q.52 CODE (6)

		Top Plate		Bottom Plate	
		Yes	No	Yes	No
55. Do you usually wear your top plate (bottom plate) when you . . .	go out	1	2	1	2
INDIVIDUAL PROMPT	are eating	1	2	1	2
	are about the house ...	1	2	1	2

	Top Plate	Bottom Plate	
56. Why don't you wear your top plate (bottom plate) all the time?			Check other plate. Go to Q.63 for this plate.

130

FOR PLATES WORN ALL DAYTIME Q.52 CODE (5)

		Top Plate	Bottom Plate
Some people are fortunate with the fit of their dentures while others are not:			
57. Do you have any difficulties with your top plate (bottom plate) when you yawn?	Difficulties	1*	1*
	Not	2	2
58. Do you have any difficulties with your top plate (bottom plate) when you are talking?	Difficulties	1*	1*
	Not	2	2
59. Would you have any difficulties with your top plate (bottom plate) if you were chewing meat?	Difficulties	1*	1*
	Not	2	2
60. Would you have any difficulties with your top plate (bottom plate) if you were to bite into a raw apple?	Difficulties	1*	1*
	No	2	2
61. During the last four weeks has your top plate (bottom plate) hurt or made your mouth sore or not?	Hurt/sore	1*	1*
	Not	2	2
62. Would you say that your top plate (bottom plate) is . . .	too loose	1*	1*
	about right	2	2
RUNNING PROMPT	or too tight?	3*	3*

INTERVIEWER CHECK Q.52 AND ABOVE

63.	AT LEAST ONE CODE WITH AN ASTERISK RINGED	1	ask Q.64
	NO CODES WITH AN ASTERISK RINGED	2	Go to Q.65

You've said . . .

64. Are you planning to visit the dentist to see about your denture(s) for that or any other reason?	Planning to visit	1	
	Not	2	ask (a)

IF NOT (2)

(a) Is there any reason why you aren't planning to visit the dentist?

TO PEOPLE WHO HAVE WORN ONE OR BOTH PLATES IN LAST 4 WEEKS

NO PLATE WORN IN LAST 4 WEEKS   DNA......................   X   Go to Q.69

I'd like to talk now about cleaning dentures (false teeth)

65(a) Do zou find that it is difficult to keep false   Yes   1
      teeth clean or not?
                                                              No   2

   (b) How often do you clean your false teeth?

      ....

   (c) Do you clean your false teeth by . . .

	Yes	No	
Soaking them	1	2	see (d)
Brushing them	3	4	see (e)
Some other method ...... (SPECIFY)	5	6	

INDIVIDUAL PROMPT

   IF YES, SOAKING THEM (1)
   (d) What do you soak them in?

   IF YES, BRUSHING THEM (3)
   (e) What do you brush them with?

66. Do you use anything to help keep your top plate
     (bottom plate) in place?

	Top Plate	Bottom Plate	
Uses something.......	1	1	ask (a)
Does not	2	2	

        IF USES SOMETHING (1)
        (a) What do you use?

67. During the last four weeks have you put   Yes   1
     anything on your dentures or gums to prevent
     or ease soreness?   No   2

68. During the last four weeks have you taken any   Yes   1
     tablets or lozenges to ease soreness?
                                                       No   2

132

TO ALL WHO HAVE EVER HAD DENTURES

		Top Plate	Bottom Plate
69.	How long ago did you get your present top plate (bottom plate)?		
	Less than a year	1	1
	1 year, less than 2 years	2	2
	2 years, less than 5 years	3	3
	5 years, less than 10 years	4	4
	10 years, less than 20 years	5	5
IF LOST ASK ABOUT THE PLATE THAT IS NOW LOST	20 years, or more	6	6

			Top Plate	Bottom Plate	
70.	Did you get your present top plate (bottom plate) through the National Health Service or did you pay for if privately?	N.H.S.	1	1	
		Private	2	2	ask (a)
		Before N.H.S.	3	3	
		Other (SPECIFY)	4	4	

IF PRIVATE (2)
(a) What was the main reason for you getting your top plate (bottom plate) privately?

71.

DNA

72.

DNA

73. Thinking about your present dentures how satisfied are (were) you with their appearance; are (were) you . . .	very satisfied	1	go to Q.74
	fairly satisfied	2	
RUNNING PROMPT	not very satisfied	3	ask (a)
	or not at all satisfied?	4	
	Informant says DNA	5	go to Q.74

IF CODE (2, 3 or 4)
(a) You say you are (were) .... rather than very satisfied. What is it about their appearance that you are (were) not completely satisfied with?

INTERVIEWER OBSERVE:
IF INFORMANT IS NOT WEARING TEETH AT TIME OF INTERVIEW—

	DNA	5	go to Q.83
74(a) Some people who wear dentures don't like their family to see them without their teeth. How much does this worry you: very much, to some extent or not at all?	Very much	1	
	To some extent	2	
	Not at all	3	
	No family	4	
(b) If people other than the family were to see you without your teeth how much would this worry you: very much, to some extent or not at all?	Very much	1	
	To some extent	2	
	Not at all	3	

Questions 75–82 DNA

---

83. When you first had dentures fitted did the dentist give you any advice on how to chew with dentures?	Advice on chewing	1
	None	2
	Can't remember	3

---

84. Did the dentist give you any advice on how to bite with the front teeth of your dentures?	Advice on biting	1
	None	2
	Can't remember	3
	Informant says DNA	4

85. Did the dentist talk to you at all about the length of time it would take you to get used to your dentures?

Yes, talked...................... 1   ask (a)

Did not 2

Can't remember 3

      IF YES, TALKED (1)
(a) How long did he say it would take you to get used to them?

---

86. Did the dentist tell you how long you should expect your dentures to last?

Yes 1

No............................. 2

Can't remember 3

---

87. When you first had your dentures did the dentist or any of his staff tell you how to clean them?

Yes, told 1

No............................. 2

Can't remember 3

---

88. Did the dentist advise you about wearing your dentures at night?

Advised 1   ask (a)

Did not 2

Can't remember 3

      IF ADVISED (1)
(a) Did he advise you to keep them in at night or to take them out?

Keep them in 1

Take them out 2

Other (SPECIFY) 3

---

89. Would you have liked the dentist to have given you some (more) advice on managing dentures?

Liked (more) advice 1

Would not...................... 2

---

90. (Can I just check) when you first had dentures fitted did the dentist or any of his staff give you a leaflet about wearing dentures?

Given leaflet 1

Not 2

Can't remember 3

---

91. When you first had partial dentures about how long did it take you to get used to having them?

92. Coping with new dentures is always strange at first. Was there anything in particular about wearing dentures that you hadn't expected?

Something unexpected 1

Not 2   ask (a)

IF SOMETHING UNEXPECTED (1)
(a) What was it?

93. Since you've had partial dentures have you enjoyed your food . . .

      RUNNING PROMPT

more than before 1

about the same as before 2

or less than before you had them? 3

94. Since you've had partial dentures have you had to change the kind of food you eat?

Had to change 1   ask (a–b)

Not 2

IF HAD TO CHANGE (1)
(a) What can you eat now that you couldn't eat before?

Nothing 1

(b) What could you eat before that you can't eat now?

Nothing 1

95. Since having partial dentures have you had any trouble with your natural teeth which you feel is connected with having dentures?

Had trouble.................... 1   ask (a)

Not 2

IF HAD TROUBLE (1)
(a) What trouble have you had?

96.

              DNA

97. If you knew someone who thought they might soon have to have a partial denture for the first time what advice would you give them?

136

DNA

		Top Plate	Bottom Plate	
99. Since you first had dentures how many top plates (bottom plates) have you had altogether?	One plate only	1	1	
	Number			ask (a–b)

IF MORE THAN ONE TOP PLATE (BOTTOM PLATE)

		Top Plate	Bottom Plate	
(a) When you had false teeth for the first time what combination of dentures did you have: a top plate only, a bottom plate only or both?	Top plate only		1	
	Bottom plate only		2	
	Both		3	

		Top Plate	Bottom Plate	
(b) Was your first top plate (bottom plate) a full plate or not?	Full plate	1	1	
	Partial..............	2	2	ask (c)
IF PARTIAL (2)				
(c) Did the top plate (bottom plate) have some front teeth on it or were they all back teeth?	Some front teeth	1	1	
	All back teeth	2	2	

100. How old were you when you first had some false teeth?	Age in years		

101. Were your first false teeth mainly for the sake of appearance or mainly to help you to eat?	Mainly for sake of appearance	1	
	Mainly to help you to eat	2	

147. Since you had your first set of dentures how many more of your own teeth have you lost?	Number lost		

TO PEOPLE WHO HAVE HAD MORE THAN ONE TOP PLATE
(BOTTOM PLATE) (SEE Q.99)

DNA: One plate only   X   go to Q.149

148. You say you've had .... top plates (bottom plates). Were any of the top plate (bottom plate) replacements needed because . . .	Top Plate Yes	Top Plate No/DK	Bottom Plate Yes	Bottom Plate No/DK
INDIVIDUAL PROMPT				
(i) you'd had more teeth taken out	1	2	1	2
(ii) the previous plate hurt or caused ulcers	1	2	1	2
(iii) the previous plate was worn down, damaged or broken	1	2	1	2
(iv) the previous plate didn't fit properly	1	2	1	2
(v) the previous plate didn't look right	1	2	1	2
(vi) the previous plate didn't match the other plate	1	2	1	2
(vii) other (SPECIFY)	1	2	1	2

149. Are there any other comments you would like to make about your teeth or dentures?

CLASSIFICATION — TO ALL

		Day	Month	Year
150. (a) Date of birth of informant				

(b) Sex of informant

Male	1
Female	2

(c) Age informant finished full time education

14 years or less	4
15 years	5
16 years	6
17 years	7
18 years or more	8
Still in f/t education	9

(d) Employment status of informant

Full time	1
Part time	2
Not in employment	3

(e) Marital status of informant

Married	1
Single	2
W/S/D	3

(f) What is the occupation of the informant?
(GIVE OCCUPATION AND INDUSTRY)

(g) IS THE INFORMANT HOH OR NOT?

Informant HOH	1	go to Q.152
Not	2	go to Q.151

---

151. What is the occupation of the HOH?
(GIVE OCCUPATION AND INDUSTRY)

INTRODUCE AS NECESSARY

152. (a) Grateful for their help—asking for a little more in order to complete the picture.

(b) Some things only a dentist looking at your teeth would see.

(c) Asking anybody who has some teeth if dentist can come back in a few days time.

(d) He won't comment on your teeth at all, to you or anyone else (ethics).

(e) Result will help to estimate the need for treatment.

(f) Reassurance that it will not hurt at all, and interviewer will be there.

(g) Length of time for examination.

Willing to have examination ...... | 1 | see (h)

Not .... | 2 | see (j)

IF WILLING (1)
(h) appointment details

GIVE INFORMANT APPOINTMENT CARD

IF NOT WILLING (2)
(j) NOTE COMMENTS

S1112

Area No.			Address No.			Person

ADULT DENTAL HEALTH
NORTHERN IRELAND 1979

Interview questionnaire 3

People with no natural teeth

Interviewer's Name .... Inf. ....

Interviewer's No. ....

			Top Plate	Bottom Plate	

51. Could I just check, have you ever had a full set of dentures or not?

Have (had) full dentures 1

Not 2   ask (a)

    IF NOT (2)

(a) Why have you never had full dentures?

GO TO Q.75

People with dentures sometimes get on better with one plate than the other so I'd like to talk about your top and bottom plates separately.

		Top Plate	Bottom Plate	
52. Have you worn your top plate (bottom plate) at all during the last four weeks?	Yes, worn	1	1	ask (a–c)
	Not	2*	2*	

    IF WORN IN LAST FOUR WEEKS (1)

(a) (Sometimes people don't get on very well with a new denture and go back to wearing their old one):

Is the top plate (bottom plate) that you wear now the most recent one you've had or not?	Wears most recent	8	8	
	Wears old one	9	9	

(I'd like to talk about the denture you wear)

(b) Do you usually keep your top plate (bottom plate) in at night?	In at night	3	3	
	Not	4	4	
(c) Do you wear your top plate (bottom plate) from the time you get up to when you go to bed?	All daytime	5	5	
	Not	6*	6*	

FOR PLATES NOT WORN IN LAST FOUR WEEKS Q.52 CODE (2)

		Top Plate	Bottom Plate	
53. Have you still got your top plate (bottom plate)?	Still got	1	1	ask (a)
	Not	2	2	ask (b)

    IF STILL GOT (1)

(a) Why don't you wear your top plate (bottom plate)?

    IF NOT (2)

(b) What happened to your top plate (bottom plate)?

INTERVIEWER

    FOR PLATES NOT WORN IN LAST FOUR WEEKS (2) ASK Q'S 53–54.

    FOR PLATES NOT WORN ALL DAYTIME (6) ASK Q'S 55–56.

    FOR PLATES WORN ALL DAYTIME (5) ASK Q'S 57–62.

54. Have you ever had a top plate (bottom plate) that you could wear?		Top		Bottom		
Had plate..........		1		1		Check other plate. Go to Q.63 for this plate.
Not		2		2		

Check other plate. Go to Q.63 for this plate.

FOR PLATES NOT WORN ALL DAYTIME Q.52 CODE (6)

55. Do you usually wear your top plate (bottom plate) when you . . .

		Top Plate		Bottom Plate	
		Yes	No	Yes	No
	go out	1	2	1	2
INDIVIDUAL PROMPT	are eating	1	2	1	2
	are about the house ...	1	2	1	2

56. Why don't you wear your top plate (bottom plate) all the time?

Top Plate	Bottom Plate	
		Check other plate. Go to Q.63 for this plate.

FOR PLATES WORN ALL DAYTIME Q.52 CODE (5)

Some people are fortunate with the fit of their dentures while others are not:

		Top Plate	Bottom Plate
57. Do you have any difficulties with your top plate (bottom plate) when you yawn?	Difficulties	1*	1*
	Not	2	2
58. Do you have any difficulties with your top plate (bottom plate) when you are talking?	Difficulties	1*	1*
	Not	2	2
59. Would you have any difficulties with your top plate (bottom plate) if you were chewing meat?	Difficulties	1*	1*
	Not	2	2
60. Would you have any difficulties with your top plate (bottom plate) if you were to bite into a raw apple?	Difficulties	1*	1*
	No	2	2
61. During the last four weeks has your top plate (bottom plate) hurt or made your mouth sore or not?	Hurt/sore	1*	1*
	Not	2	2
62. Would you say that your top plate (bottom plate) is . . .	too loose	1*	1*
	about right	2	2
RUNNING PROMPT	or too tight?	3*	3*

INTERVIEWER CHECK Q.52 AND ABOVE

63.			
AT LEAST ONE CODE WITH AN ASTERISK RINGED		1	ask Q.64
NO CODES WITH AN ASTERISK RINGED		2	Go to Q.65

You've said . . .

64. Are you planning to visit the dentist to see about your denture(s) for that or any other reason?

Planning to visit   1

¹ot   2   ask (a)

IF NOT (2)

(a) Is there any reason why you aren't planning to visit the dentist?

TO PEOPLE WHO HAVE WORN ONE OR BOTH PLATES IN LAST 4 WEEKS

NEITHER PLATE WORN IN LAST 4 WEEKS   DNA   X   Go to Q.69

I'd like to talk now about cleaning dentures (false teeth)

65(a) Do you find that it is difficult to keep false teeth clean or not?

Yes   1

No   2

(b) How often do you clean your false teeth?

. . . .

(c) Do you clean your false teeth by . . .

INDIVIDUAL PROMPT

	Yes	No	
Soaking them	1	2	see (d)
Brushing them	3	4	see (e)
Some other method . . . . . . (SPECIFY)	5	6	

IF YES, SOAKING THEM (1)
(d) What do you soak them in?

IF YES, BRUSHING THEM (3)
(e) What do you brush them with?

66. Do you use anything to help keep your top plate (bottom plate) in place?

	Top Plate	Bottom Plate	
Uses something	1	1	ask (a)
Does not	2	2	

IF USES SOMETHING (1)
(a) What do you use?

143

		Top Plate	Bottom Plate
67. During the last four weeks have you put anything on your dentures or gums to prevent or ease soreness?	Yes .... 1 No 2		
68. During the last four weeks have you taken any tablets or lozenges to ease soreness?	Yes .... 1 No 2		

TO ALL WHO HAVE EVER HAD DENTURES

	Top Plate	Bottom Plate	
69. How long ago did you get your present top plate (bottom plate)?			
Less than a year	1		
1 year, less than 2 years	2	2	
2 years, less than 5 years	3	3	
5 years, less than 10 years	4	4	
10 years, less than 20 years	5	5	
IF LOST ASK ABOUT THE PLATE THAT IS NOW LOST 20 years, or more	6	6	
70. Did you get your present top plate (bottom plate) through the National Health Service or did you pay for if privately? N.H.S.	1	1	
Private	2	2	ask (a)
Before N.H.S.	3	3	
Other (SPECIFY)	4	4	

IF PRIVATE (2)

(a) What was the main reason for you getting your top plate (bottom plate) privately?

71. Do you know how much it would cost you nowadays to have a full set of false teeth under the National Health Service?	Yes .... 1 No 2		ask (a)

IF YES (1)

(a) How much does it cost?

72. How many full top plates (bottom plates) have you had since the last of your natural teeth were taken out?

	Top Plate	Bottom Plate	
1	1	1	go to Q.73
2	2	2	
3	3	3	
4	4	4	ask (a)
5 or more	5	5	

IF 2 OR MORE (2, 3, 4 or 5)
(a) Were any of your top plate (bottom plate) replacements needed because the previous plate . . .

INDIVIDUAL PROMPT

	Top Plate		Bottom Plate	
	Yes	No/DK	Yes	No/DK
(i) hurt or caused ulcers...................	1	2	1	2
(ii) was worn down, damaged or broken	1	2	1	2
(iii) didn't fit properly......................	1	2	1	2
(iv) didn't look right	1	2	1	2
(v) didn't match the other plate	1	2	1	2
(vi) other (SPECIFY)	1	2	1	2

73. Thinking about your present dentures how satisfied are (were) you with their appearance; are (were) you . . .

RUNNING PROMPT

very satisfied	1	
fairly satisfied	2	
not very satisfied	3	ask (a)
or not at all satisfied?...........	4	

IF CODE (2, 3 or 4)
(a) You say you are (were) .... rather than very satisfied. What is it about their appearance that you are (were) not completely satisfied with?

INTERVIEWER OBSERVE:
IF INFORMANT IS NOT WEARING TEETH AT TIME OF INTERVIEW—

DNA...........................	5	go to Q.75

74(a) Some people who wear dentures don't like their family to see them without their teeth.
How much does this worry you: very much, to some extent or not at all?

Very much....................	1
To some extent	2
Not at all.....................	3
No family	4

(b) If people other than the family were to see you without your teeth how much would this worry you: very much, to some extent or to some extent or not at all?

Very much	1
To some extent	2
Not at all.....................	3

145

TO ALL

I'd like to talk now about when you had the last of your natural teeth out.

75.	How many years ago did you have the of your own teeth taken out?	Up to 5 years ago	1
		Over 5 up to 10 years ago	2
		Over 10 up to 15 years ago	3
	PROMPT AS NECESSARY	Over 15 up to 20 years ago	4
		Over 20 up to 30 years ago	5
		Over 30 years ago	6	ask (a)
	IF OVER 30 YEARS AGO (6)		
	(a) Was this before or after 1948 when the National Health Service began?	Before	1
		After	2

76.	How old were you when you lost the last of your natural teeth?	Age in years	

77.	When you lost the last of your own teeth many teeth were there to be taken out altogether?	1–11	1
		12–20	2
		21 or more	3

	IF ONLY ONE TOOTH TAKEN OUT RING CODE (1)		
78.	Were these all taken out together or were they taken out over a series of visits?	All in one visit	1
		Series of visits	2

79.	Why did the last of your own teeth have to be taken out, was it because . . .	the teeth were decayed	1
		the gums were bad	2
	CODE ALL THAT APPLY	or was it for some other reason... (SPECIFY)	3

80.	Did you find losing the last of your natural teeth and having full dentures . . .	very upsetting	1
		a little upsetting	2
		or not at all upsetting?..........	3

81.	Did you suggest to the dentist that the last of your natural teeth should come out or did he suggest this to you?	Informant suggested to dentist	1
		Dentist suggested to informant	2
		Other (SPECIFY)	3

	TO ALL WHO HAVE EVER HAD FULL DENTURES Q.51 (1)		
		DNA: Never had full dentures	X	go to Q.95
82.	How long after you had the last of your own teeth out did you have false teeth in, was it . . .	the same day...................	1
		up to 1 month	2
	RUNNING PROMPT	more than 1 month up to 3 months	3
		more than 3 months up to 6 months	4
		or more than 6 months later?	5

146

83.	When you first had full dentures did the dentist give you any advice on how to chew with dentures?	Advice on chewing	1
		None	2
		Can't remember	3
84.	Did the dentist give you any advice on how to bite with the front teeth of your dentures?	Advice on bitino	1
		None	2
		Can't remember	3
		Informant says DNA	4
85.	Did the dentist talk to you at all about the length of time it would take you to get used to your dentures? IF YES, TALKED (1) (a) How long did he say it would take you to get used to them?	Yes, talked....................	1 ask (a)
		Did not	2
		Can't remember	3
86.	Did the dentist tell you how long you should expect your dentures to last?	Yes	1
		No	2
		Can't remember	3
87.	When you first had your dentures did the dentist or any of his staff tell you how to clean them?	Yes, told	1
		No	2
		Can't remember	3
88.	Did the dentist advise you about wearing your dentures at night? IF ADVISED (1) (a) Did he advise you to keep them in at night or to take them out?	Advised	1 ask (a)
		Did not	2
		Can't remember	3
		Keep thm in	1
		Take them out	2
		Other (SPECIFY)	3
89.	Would you have liked the dentist to have given you some (more) advice on managing dentures?	Liked (more) advice	1
		Would not	2
90.	(Can I just check) when you first had full dentures did the dentist or any of his staff give you a leaflet about wearing dentures?	Given leaflet	1
		Not	2
		Can't remember	3

91. When you first had full dentures about how long
     did it take you to get used to having them?

---

92. Coping with new dentures is always strange at
     first. Was there anything in particular about
     wearing dentures that you hadn't expected?

     Something unexpected 1

     Not 2   ask (a)

          IF SOMETHING UNEXPECTED (1)
     (a) What was it?

---

93. Since you've had full dentures
     have you enjoyed your food . . .

     more than before 1

     about the same as before 2

     or less than before you had them? 3

---

94. Since you've had full dentures have
     you had to change the kind of food you eat?

     Had to change 1   ask (a–b)

     Not 2

          IF HAD TO CHANGE (1)
     (a) What can you eat now that you
          couldn't eat before?

     Nothing 1

     (b) What could you eat before that you
          can't eat now?

     Nothing 1

TO ALL

95. Thinking about when you lost the last of your natural teeth
     can you tell me a little more about how you felt?

---

96. Did you expect to lose your teeth around then
     or were you surprised to have them out at
     that age?

     Expected to lose................. 1

     Surprised at that age 2

     Other (SPECIFY) 3

148

97. If you knew someone who thought they might soon have to have the rest of their teeth out and full dentures fitted what advice would you give them?

(We've been talking about full dentures but, of course) people may have partial dentures (some false teeth) before they lose all their own teeth.

| 98. When you had the last of your own teeth out had you previously had any dentures? | Previously had dentures .... | 1 | ask (a) |
| | Did not .... | 2 | go to Q.115 |

IF PREVIOUSLY HAD DENTURES (1)

(a) What kind of dentures did you have, a top plate only, a bottom plate only or both?	Top plate only	1	ask (b)
	Bottom plate only	2	ask (c)
	Both	3	ask (b–c)

IF TOP PLATE OR BOTH (1 or 3)

| (b) Was the top plate a full plate or not? | Full top plate .... | 1 |
| | Partial...................... | 2 |

IF BOTTOM PLATE OR BOTH (2 or 3)

| (c) Was the bottom plate a full plate or not? | Full bottom plate.............. | 1 |
| | Partial...................... | 2 |

| 99. ⌈Was that top plate (bottom plate)⌉ ⌊Were those plates⌋ the only partial denture(s) you'd had or had you previously had other dentures? | One set only .... | 1 | go to Q.100 |
| | Had others .... | 2 | ask (a) |

IF HAD OTHERS (2)

(a) When you had dentures for the very first time what did you have, a top plate only, a bottom plate only or both?	Top plate only	1	ask (b)
	Bottom plate only	2	ask (c)
	Both	3	ask (b–c)

IF TOP PLATE OR BOTH (1 or 3)

| (b) Was the top plate a full plate or not? | Full top plate .... | 1 |
| | Partial...................... | 2 |

IF BOTTOM PLATE OR BOTH (2 or 3)

| (c) Was the bottom plate a full plate or not? | Full bottom plate.............. | 1 |
| | Partial...................... | 2 |

| 100. How old were you when you first had some false teeth? | Age in years .... | .... |

| 101. Were your first false teeth mainly for the sake of appearance or mainly to help you to eat? | Mainly for sake of appearance .... | 1 |
| | Mainly to help you to eat .... | 2 |

115. Different people have different ideas as to what things help to keep teeth healthy. I'd like to talk to you about some things people have mentioned. Can you tell me how important you consider them for keeping natural teeth healthy?

SHOW CARD A

Would you say that . . .

	FOR KEEPING NATURAL TEETH HEALTHY				
	very important	fairly important	not very important	not at all important	D.K.
(i) Not eating sweets is	1	2	3	4	5
(ii) Regular visits to the dentist are	1	2	3	4	5
(iii) Cleaning teeth regularly is	1	2	3	4	5
(iv) Having fluoride in the water is	1	2	3	4	5

116.   DNA

I'd like to talk now about your childhood dental experiences.

117. When you were a child how much encouragement were you given to clean your teeth. Were you given . . .

RUNNING PROMPT

a great deal	1
a fair amount	2
not much	3
or no encouragement at all	4

118. When you were a child (that is before you were 16) did you ever go to a dentist?

Went to a dentist	1	ask (a)
Did not	2	go to Q.119

IF WENT TO A DENTIST (1)
(a) Did you go to the school dentist, some other dentist or both?

School dentist	1	ask (c–d)
Other dentist	2	
Both	3	ask (b–d)

IF OTHER DENTIST OR BOTH (2 or 3)
(b) (Excluding visits to the school dentist) as a child did you go to the dentist for . . .

RUNNING PROMPT

a regular check up	1
an occasional check up	2
or only when you were having trouble with your teeth?	3
Other (SPECIFY)	4

150

Thinking about any treatment you had then:

(c) Did you have any teeth filled before were 16?

Teeth filled	1
Not	2
DK/can't remember.............	3

(d) Did you have any teeth taken out before you were 16?

Teeth taken out	1
Not	2
DK/can't remember.............	3

(We've talked a little about childhood and) now I'd like to talk about the dental experiences you've had through the whole of your life.

IF TEETH FILLED WHEN CHILD (Q.118 (c) CODE (1)) RING (1) AND ASK (a–b).

119. Have you ever had any teeth filled?

Teeth filled	1	ask (a–b)
Not	2	

IF TEETH FILLED (1)

(a) Have you ever had an injection in your gum to kill the pain of a filling?

Injection in gum.................	1
Not	2

(b) Have you ever had an injection in your arm to kill the pain of a filling?

Injection in arm	1
Not	2

120(a) Have you ever had gas to have teeth taken out?

Had gas	1
Not	2

(b) Have you ever had an injection in your gum to have teeth taken out?

Injection in gum.................	1
Not	2

(c) Have you ever had an injection in your arm to have teeth taken out?

Injection in arm	1
Not	2

121. Have you ever had an X-ray taken of your teeth?

Had X-ray.....................	1
Not	2

122. While you had your own teeth did you go to the dentist for regular checks ups, occasional check ups or only when you had trouble with your teeth?

Regular check ups	1
Occasional check ups	2
Only when had trouble with teeth .	3

Questions 123–127 DNA

I'd like to talk now about going to the dentist.

128. Have you been to the dentist in the last year?

Yes	1	ask (a)
No	2	ask (b)

IF YES (1)

(a) (Can I just check) are you in the middle of a course of treatment now or not?

In middle of treatment	1	go to Q.129
Not	2	

IF NO (2)

(b) About how long ago was your last visit the dentist?

PROMPT AS NECESSARY

More than 1 up to 2 years ago ...	1	ask (d)
More than 2 up to 3 years ago ...	2	go to Q.129
More than 3 up to 5 years ago ...	3	
More than 5 up to 10 years ago ..	4	
More than 10 up to 15 years ago .	5	go to Q.145
More than 15 up to 20 years ago .	6	
More than 20 years ago	7	ask (c)

IF LAST WENT TO DENTIST MORE THAN 20 YEARS AGO (7)

(c) Was your last visit to the dentist since 1948 or before 1948?

1948 or since	1	go to Q.145
Before 1948	2	

IF MORE THAN 1 UP TO 2 YEARS AGO (b) CODE (1)

(d) Was your last visit before or after 1 September 1978?

Before April 1st	1
April 1st or after	2

129. The last time you went to the dentist what was it that made you go?

130. For the treatment you needed at that time how many visits did you make to the dentist?

One visit	1
Two visits	2
Three visits	3
Four visits	4
Five or more visits	5

131. (Can I just check) during the visit(s) you made to the dentist for that course of treatment did you have . . .

INDIVIDUAL PROMPT

	YES	NO	D.K.
Any X-rays taken	1	2	3
Any teeth extracted	1	2	3
Fitting of new dentures	1	2	3
Repair of old dentures	1	2	3
Any other treatment (SPECIFY)	1	2	3

132.	Was your treatment under the Health Service, was it private or was it something else?	National Health Service	1	
		Private	2	ask (b)
		N.H.S. and private	3	ask (a–b)
		Community Dental Service	4	
		Armed Forces	5	
	....	Other (SPECIFY)	6	

IF NHS AND PRIVATE (3)

(a) What treatment did you have privately?

IF ANY PRIVATE (2 or 3)

(b) What was the main reason for you having this treatment done privately?

SEE EXTRA QUESTION—N.I. QUESTIONS

133.	How much did the treatment cost you?	Cost (SPECIFY)	1	ask (a)
		Nothing	2	ask (b)
	....	DK	3	go to Q.134

IF PAID FOR TREATMENT (1)

(a) Did the treatment cost more than you expected, about what you expected or less than you expected	More than expected	1	
	About what expected	2	
	Less than expected	3	go to Q.134
	Other (SPECIFY)	4	

IF NOTHING (2)

(b) Why didn't it cost you anything?	No treatment...................	1	go to Q. 134
PROMPT AS NEC.	Under 21, pregnant or nursing mother	2	
	Other (SPECIFY)...............	3	ask (c)

(c) When you went to the dentist did you expect the treatment would be free?	Yes	1	
	No	2	

134.	Thinking about the dental practice you went to for your last treatment, was that the first time you had been to that dentist or group of dentists or had you been there before?	First time......................	1	ask (d)
		Been before	2	ask (a–d)

IF BEEN BEFORE (2)

(a) For about how many years have you been going to that dentist or group of dentists?	Less than a year	1	
	One year less than two..........	2	
	Two years less than five.........	3	
	Five years or more	4	
	DK/can't remember.............	5	

153

(d) Last time you wanted to see the dentist about how long did you have to wait for an appointment?

135. How did you come to choose that particular dentist?

Can't remember 9

USE PROMPTS

136. In the last five years have you had any difficulty in getting any treatment under the National Health Service?

Had difficulty 1   ask (a–b)

Not 2

    IF HAD DIFFICULTY (1)
(a) What treatment couldn't you get?

        PART OF IT/
        PART OF IT
        IF PART WHAT PART?

(b) What did you do about it?

Questions 137 and 138 DNA

154

I'd like to talk now about going to the dentist.

I'd like to talk generally now about the cost of dental treatment under the Health Service.

139. When you go to the dentist to have treatment do you normally have some idea of how much it's going to cost you?	Has some idea		1
	Does not	2	

140. Do you know where you can find out about Health Service dental charges?	Yes	1	ask (a)
	No............................	2	
IF YES (1)			
(a) Where can you find out?	Dentist	1	
	G.P.O.	2	
	Other (SPECIFY)	3	

141. When you have to pay at the dentist does he usually tell you what the total cost is made up of?	Yes	1	
	No............................	2	
	Never paid	3	

142. I'd like you to look at these different treatments and tell me how much you think each would cost, whether it would cost nothing or whether it would cost £2 or less, between £2 and £5, or £5 or more?

SHOW CARDS B AND C	TREATMENT WOULD COST				
COURSE OF TREATMENT (B)	Nothing (Free)	£2 or less	Between £2 and £5	£5 or more	D.K.
Exam, 2 teeth out	1	2	3	4	5
Exam, 1 large filling, 1 tooth out...............	1	2	3	4	5
Examination only	1	2	3	4	5
Exam, 2 X-rays, scale and polish, 1 sall filling	1	2	3	4	5
Exam, 4 teeth out, new dentures fitted	1	2	3	4	5
Exam, 2 X-rays, 6 teeth out, gas	1	2	3	4	5
Repair of cracked denture	1	2	3	4	5
Exam, 2 X-rays, scale and polish	1	2	3	4	5

155

143. For most kinds of treatment under the Health Service the patient pays the full cost up to the first £7.

(a) As a maximum charge do you think £7 is:

RUNNING PROMPT

too high	1
about right	2
or too low?	3

(b) A few kinds of dental treatment are rather expensive and so the patient has to pay more than £7 to be treated under the Health Service.

Do you know what kinds of treatment cost the patient more than £7?

Yes	1	ask (c)
No	2	

IF YES (1)

(c) What kinds of treatment cost the patient more than £7?

144. Some people get exemption from dental charges so that all the treatment they have is free.
Do you know what kinds of people get free treatment?

Yes	1	ask (a)
No	2	

IF YES (1)

(a) What kinds of people get free treatment?

Pregnant or nursing mothers	1
Other (SPECIFY)	2

TO ALL

145. People have mentioned all sorts of things that make them put off going to the dentist. Can you look at this card and tell me for each of the statements I read out whether these things apply to you very much, a fair amount, not very much or not at all.

SHOW CARD D	APPLIES TO ME				
I put off going to the dentist because . . .	very much	à fair amount	not very much	not at all	D.K.
I'm scared of the dentist	1	2	3	4	5
It's difficult to get time off work	1	2	3	4	5
It's too expensive to go too often	1	2	3	4	5
I haven't got a regular dentist	1	2	3	4	5
I can't be bothered really	1	2	3	4	5
It's difficult to get an appointment...........	1	2	3	4	5
It's a long way to go	1	2	3	4	5

156

146. What do you find most unpleasant about going to the dentist?

GO TO N.I. QUESTIONS

147. Are there any other comments you would like to make about having false teeth?

CLASSIFICATION — TO ALL

	Day	Month	Year
150. (a) Date of birth of informant			

(b) Sex of informant

Male 1

Female 2

(c) Age informant finished full time education

14 years or less 4

15 years 5

16 years 6

17 years 7

18 years or more 8

Still in f/t education 9

(d) Employment status of informant

Full time 1

Part time 2

Not in employment 3

(e) Marital status of informant

Married 1

Single 2

W/S/D........................ 3

(f) What is the occupation of the informant?
(GIVE OCCUPATION AND INDUSTRY)

(g) IS THE INFORMANT HOH OR NOT?

Informant HOH 1

Not 2   go to Q.151

157

151. What is the occupation of the HOH?
(GIVE OCCUPATION AND INDUSTRY)

ADDITIONAL QUESTIONS FOR NORTHERN IRELAND SURVEY

Please ask the first question below on private dental treatment as Question 32(c) on the yellow or pink schedules, or Question 132(c) on the green schedule.

32(c) IF HAD ALL OR SOME TREATMENT DONE PRIVATELY.

Did you want to have this treatment done privately, or would you have preferred to have on the NHS?	Wanted it done privately 1		return to main schedule
	Would have preferred NHS.......	2	ask (a)
(a) Did you ask the dentist if he would do this treatment on the NHS, or not?	Yes, asked	1	
	No	2	
(b) Were you given any reasons for not being able to have the treatment done on the NHS, or not?	Yes	1	ask (i)
	No...........................	2	return to main schedule
(i) What reasons were you given?			
			return to main schedule

ATTITUDES TO AVAILABILITY OF DENTAL SERVICES

Q.1 (a) Would you say that it is usually	very easy	1	ask Q.2
	fairly easy	2	ask Q.2
	fairly difficult	3	ask (b)
	very difficult	4	ask (b)
	don't know/no opinion...........	8	ask Q.2
for you to obtain health service dental treatment from your dentist?			
(b) What makes it difficult? (Specify)			

Q.2 Approximately how far is the dentist's surgery from your home? Is it	less than a mile	1	
	1 mile, less than 2	2	
	2 mile, less than 5	3	
	5 miles, less than 10	4	
	more than 10 miles/specify?	5	
	don't know, can't estimate	8	Q.3

159

Q.3	If you were going to the dentist's from home, how would you usually get there?	walk all the way	1	
		go by public transport	2	
		drive yourself by car/motorbike ...	3	
		be driven by someone else	4	
		bicycle	5	
		other (specify)	6	Q.4

Q.4	About how long would it take you to get to the dentist's surgery from home if you were (Specify means of transport at Q.3)?	about 5 mins	1	
		about 10 mins	2	
		about 15 mins	3	
		about 20 mins	4	
		more than 20 mins (Specify)	5	
		don't know/can't say	8	Q.5

Q.5	On the whole, how convenient is the dental surgery which you attend? Is it	very convenient	1	
		fairly convenient	2	
		fairly inconvenient	3	
		very inconvenient	4	
		can't say/don't know	8	Introduction

Introduction
I would like to ask you several questions about any occasions when you have tried to get emergency dental treatment.

Q.6	In the last 5 years, have there been any occasions when you tried to see a dentist outside normal surgery hours, because you were having trouble with your teeth and needed treatment urgently?	Yes	1	Ask (a)
		No	2	go to Q.14
		DK	3	
	(a) When was the last time you wanted to see a dentist outside normal surgery hours?	Less than a year ago	1	
		1 year but less than 2 years ago ..	2	
		2 years but less than 5 years ago .	3	
		DK/Can't remember	4	

Q.7	On that occasion, what was the matter?			
				Q.8

160

Q.8	How soon after the trouble started did you try to see a dentist?	Same day	1	
		Next day	2	
		2–3 days later	3	
		4–6 days later	4	
		1 week later, or more	5	
		DK/Can't remember	6	Q.9
Q.9	Was it a weekday, a Saturday or a Sunday when you tried to see a dentist for treatment?	Weekday	1	
		Saturday	2	
		Sunday	3	
		Bank Holiday	4	
	(a) What time was it when you tried to see a dentist?	9.01–12.00	1	
		12.01–18.00	2	
		18.01–20.00	3	
		20.01– 9.00	4	
		DK/Can't remember	5	Q.10
Q.10	Which dentist did you try to see? Was it . . .	an ordinary dental surgeon	1	ask (a)
	RUNNING PROMPT	or a dentist at a hospital?	2	go to Q.11
	(a) Was that a dentist you had been to before, or not?	Yes	1	
		No	2	
Q.11	Did you eventually succeed in getting the treatment done by that dentist?	Yes	1	ask (a)
		No	2	go to Q.12
	(a) How long after you first tried, did you succeed in getting the treatment done?	The same day	1	
		The next day	2	
		2–3 days later	3	ask (b)
		4–5 days later	4	
		More than 5 days later	5	
		DK/Can't remember	6	go to Q.14
	(b) How satisfied were you with the time you waited to get the treatment done? Would you say you were . . . RUNNING PROMPT	very satisfied	1	
		fairly satisfied	2	go to Q.14
		fairly dissatisfied	3	
		or very dissatisfied?	4	
Q.12	Why were you unable to see that dentist?	DK/No idea	1	
				Q.13

161

Q.13 Did you do anything else at the time to try to get the necessary treatment done, or did you just wait to see the dentist in normal surgery hours?	Yes, did something else	1	ask (a) & (b)
	No, just waited	2	ask (b)
(a) What else did you do?			
(b) So, how long after you first tried did you succeed in getting the necessary treatment done?	The same day	1	
	The next day	2	
	2–3 days later	3	ask (c)
	4–5 days later	4	
	More than 5 days later	5	
	DK/Can't remember	6	go to introduction
(c) How satisfied were you with the time you waited to get the treatment done? Would you say you were . . .	very satisfied	1	
	fairly satisfied	2	
RUNNING PROMPT	fair dissatisfied	3	go to introduction
	or very dissatisfied?	4	

Introduction

Dentists work in different types of setting and I would like to ask you one or two questions about your views on these (ask Q.14).

Q.14 There are three types of dental service available for children. (Show Card).			
Which of these dental services would you prefer for children?	Mobile caravan dental clinic visiting schools	1	
	Children visiting school clinic	2	
	Children visiting a health service dentist in his own surgery	3	
	Don't know/no opinion	8	Q.15

Q.15 The three branches of the dental service are:

(i) the general dental service eg dentists working in their own surgeries;

(ii) the community dental service eg the school dental service and the dental service for the housebound or handicapped;

(iii) the hospital dental service eg dentists working in hospitals.

We are interested in finding out how satisfactory a service dentists are providing in these areas.

Firstly

The general dental service	satisfactory	1	
	not satisfactory	2	
	don't know/no opinion	8	

The school dental service	satisfactory.....................	1	
	not satisfactory	2	
	don't know/no opinion	8	
The dental service for the housebound or handicapped	satisfactory.....................	1	
	not satisfactory	2	
	don't know/no opinion	8	
The hospital dental service	satisfactory.....................	1	
	not satisfactory	2	
	don't know/no opinion	8	

Q.16   If code 2 is selected in any of the four above sections, ask:—

Why do you feel (specify particular area from above) is not satisfactory? (Specify)

INTERVIEWER: Specify both the area needing improvement **and** the improvement suggested.

Return to Question 47   (yellow)
              Question 147 (green)
              Question 149 (pink)

Whichever appropriate.

ADULT DENTAL HEALTH SURVEY
NORTHERN IRELAND — 1979

*CRITERIA FOR THE ASSESSMENT
OF DENTAL HEALTH

DEPARTMENT OF HEALTH AND SOCIAL SERVICES

SOCIAL RESEARCH DIVISION
CENTRAL ECONOMIC SERVICE
DEPARTMENT OF FINANCE

SEPTEMBER 1979

CRITERIA FOR THE DENTAL EXAMINATION

The Criteria should be studied in conjunction with the examination form. Name, Date of Birth, Sex, Serial Number and dental status will be completed by the Interviewer before entering the house.

IF THE PATIENT HAS DENTURES THEY WILL BE ASKED TO WEAR THEM FOR THIS PART OF THE EXAMINATION.

1. Existence of the Teeth

Permanent teeth will be examined in the following order:

Upper left — upper right — lower right — lower left.

Every tooth shown on the chart should be given one of the following codes (i.e. code all 32 teeth):

P — Present
M — Missing
U — Broken down tooth and definite pulp involvement
C — Crown or temporary crown.

Notes:

1. **Codes P and M.** The use of these codes, where the true designation of a tooth may be in doubt, needs some clarification. The following suggestions may help:

a. Estimate gap sizes, allowing for drifting.

b. Look behind the last standing tooth. Could there have been another tooth there?

c. Look at the tissue in spaces. Is it heaped up, indicating a considerable closure of this space already?

d. Examine the form of the tooth; eg in the upper jaw, third molars are smaller and have a less well-defined cusp pattern.

e. Look at the other quadrants.

f. Ask the patient about loss of teeth.

g. If there is doubt about the identification of the last standing tooth then score the tooth as the second molar, not as the third.

h. If there is a decidious tooth present in the arch then its successor will be scored as M.

2. **Code C.** This is FULL crown. Three-quarter crowns are coded as fillings. In this case use code **P**.

---

*The criteria used for the assessment of adult dental health in the Northern Ireland survey are identical to those defined for the United Kingdom adult dental health survey of 1978.

Acknowledgement is paid to the staff of the Social Survey Division of the Office of Population Censuses and Surveys and of the Department of Dental Health, University of Birmingham who defined the criteria and who have kindly permitted them to be used in the Northern Ireland survey of 1979.

Replacement of Missing Teeth (Gaps)

Every tooth which has been classified as M in the section above, will be additionally coded into one of the following categories:—

D — The tooth has been replaced by a denture or prosthesis which can be removed from the mouth.

B — The tooth has been replaced by a bridge or prosthesis which cannot be removed from the mouth.

N — No space.

S — Space.

Note:

Category N will be used when the remaining space is equal or less than ½ the width of the missing tooth, and for all missing third molars.

AT THIS POINT IN THE EXAMINATION THE PATIENT WILL BE ASKED TO REMOVE THEIR DENTURES.

2. Denture Bearing Areas (DBA)

(This section applies only if a denture has been worn during the last four weeks).

When the patient has removed the denture, the denture-bearing areas will be examined. The examiner will assess whether, in his opinion, the denture itself is having a destructive effect on these tissues. Only those conditions related to the wearing of partial dentures will be assessed eg gum stripping, tilting of teeth and caries on teeth adjacent to the denture. Conditions common to full or partial dentures will not be recorded eg traumatic ulcers, denture stomatitis.

The findings will be recorded separately for each denture as follows:

affecting = 1
not affecting = 2

Note: In the situation where a flabby ridge exists beneath a full upper or lower denture opposed by either natural teeth or a partial denture, this is recorded in this section as "affecting".

IF IN DOUBT, SCORE LOW.

3. Surfaces

The teeth which are present will be re-examined in the order given before. Each will be re-identified (to ensure correct recodes) and each surface coded in the order, mesial, occlusal, distal, lingual and buccal. The surfaces are recorded in the following categories:

O — The surface is sound. None of the criteria under X are applicable, and the surface is not filled. (Say "zero" rather than "nought" or "O".)

A — The surface is restored with amalgam.

G — The surface is restored with gold.

S — The surface is restored with a synthetic filling material.

X — The surface has decay present, a temporary dressing, or a missing restoration.

The surface is regarded as decayed if, in the opinion of the examiner, after visual examination, there is a carious cavity. If doubt exists it will be investigated with the probe supplied and unless the point enters the lesion the surface will be recorded as sound. (Zero).

Notes:

a. Where a surface has been restored with more than one type of filling material only code the material which occupies the largest area.

b. The code for the filling material, (chosen as in a. if necessary) may be multicoded with X. (say A **and** X).

c. Chipped or cracked fillings which need replacement are multicoded with the symbol for the major restorative material together with X.

d. Where a filling from one surface encroaches on another, eg an occlusal filling with buccal or lingual extensions, then the filling is charted as being present on all surfaces on to which it extends.

e. New caries at the junction of a filling and the tooth is charted as code X if the criteria for code X are fulfilled. This is multicoded as filling and caries.

f. With rotated teeth identify the anatomical surfaces of the tooth when coding, and not those related to its new position.

g. Do not transilluminate the molar and premolar teeth.

h. If a molar or premolar is sound say "all zero". Otherwise say zero for each sound surface.

IF IN DOUBT, SCORE LOW.

4. Periodontal Status (Gums)

Method of Assessment

In applying the scoring methods for soft deposits, calculus, gingivitis and periodontal involvement the mouth is divided into six segments, three upper and three lower, as follows: anterior, from distal surface of canine to distal surface of canine, and left and right posterior from first premolar to the last tooth in the arch, including the interdental papilla distal to the canine. Each assessment should be made independently: Debris should be noted before calculus is recorded, and all recordings of calculus should be made before those of gingivitis or periodontal involvement. The presence or absence of each of these four conditions will be recorded for the upper left posterior segment, then for the upper anterior segment, and finally for the upper right posterior segment. The opposite sequence will be followed for the lower jaw; ie the lower right segment, lower anterior segment and finally the lower left segment.

The lingual and vestibular aspect of each segment should be inspected for each assessment. All assessments in a particular segment should cease when a condition is detected on any aspect of any tooth in that segment.

Criteria for Assessment and Coding

A. *Soft Deposits:*

The only instrument to be used is a mouth mirror. If soft deposits are clearly visible to the unaided eye at the gingival margin of one or more teeth within a segment, score "1" for that segment. No attempt should be made to dry the teeth to make soft deposits more readily apparent. If no soft deposit is detected visually within a segment, score "0" for that segment.

B. *Calculus* (Supragingival)

Score "1" for a segment when calculus is obviously present in contact with the gingival margin of one or more teeth in the segment. Any obvious deposit suspected of being calculus when assessed by direct inspection or with the aid of a mouth mirror, should be tested with a periodontal probe to confirm that it is in fact calcified, and a score of "1" is then recorded. If the deposit is not calcified score "0".

C. *Gingivitis*

The state of the gums will be coded according to one of the following criteria:

0 — The gums appear healthy; pale pink and firm with no evidence of inflammation. (No treatment is indicated).

1 — Moderate gingivitis*: The gingival margin is redder and may be slightly oedematous. There is no tendency to bleed. (In this case the gingivitis should respond to plaque control alone).

2 — Intense gingivitis*: The gingivae are markedly red and oedematous. They bleed on digital pressure. (Only if doubt exists in this category should an attempt be made to elicit bleeding). (Plaque control alone may not be sufficient to resolve the condition).

Certain gingival conditions exist which, although scoring "0" or "1" on the gingivitis assessment, require more than plaque control alone to resolve the condition. These should be given the appropriate gingival score plus an asterisk and details recorded in Comments. (eg Gingival hyperplasia).

This should be recorded for each segment involved.

Mucosal trauma, due to incisors biting on the palatal gingiva or labial gingiva should be marked as an asterisk and recorded in Comments.

D. *Periodontitis*

A segment will be examined for one of or both the following conditions:

Gingivitis category 2, as defined above
Marked changes in gingival contour.

If either or both the above conditions exist, periodontitis is suspected in that segment. In this case proceed as follows:—

1. Test for definite tooth mobility. If mobility is found **Score 1,** otherwise proceed to

2. The periodontal probe is used on all tooth surfaces which fulfill the criteria for PERIODONTITIS in D to detect pockets greater in depth than 3 mm beyond the amelo-cemental junction. If such a pocket is found then **score 1** for that segment. The first mark on the periodontal probe is at 3 mm.

Note: In the case of doubt in any of the above conditions then the lower category should be recorded.

---

*Should fibrous enlargement be associated with gingivitis, the gingivitis should be recorded according to the criteria, an asterisk recorded for the appropriate segment and the condition recorded on the back of the form.

5. Crowding

Assessment of crowding is to be made on teeth erupted into the oral cavity at that time and no account taken of missing teeth and/or potential crowding. Each segment is to be recorded separately, the middle segments to include incisors and canines, and the right and left segments to include premolars and molars. Record in the following categories:—

0 — No crowding, the standing teeth fit into that segment of the dental arch without overlapping or irregularity. (Score zero if not suitable for treatment.)

1 — There is shortage of space or overlap or irregularity in that segment of not more than one premolar width (left and right segments), or one lower lateral incisor width (lower middle segment), or one upper lateral incisor width (upper middle segment).

2 — There is shortage of space or overlap or irregularity in that segment to a greater extent than in the previous category (1).

IF IN DOUBT, SCORE LOW

Occlusal Assessment

The assessment of overbite and overjet should be made only when there is sufficient posterior support for the patient to maintain a consistent occlusion and where natural incisor teeth are present. The assessment is to be made therefore with the denture out, the teeth in centric occlusion, and the Frankfort plane horizontal.

6. Overjet

This is the horizontal distance in mms between the labial surfaces of the upper and lower central incisors. The general incisor relationship should first be assessed ie if the majority are proclined then score as positive, if retroclined, score as negative, and if edge-to-edge as zero. Then a measurement should be made with the gauge supplied on the central incisor teeth with the greatest displacement in the same direction as the general displacement. When no assessment is possible, the recorded will strike through this part of the form. If the assessment falls between marks on the gauge, record the lower mark.

Note: Select the most protruded tooth for measurement. Score at the mid point of the tooth. Use the gauge horizontally. Score out this section in cases of anterior open bite. In all other cases, take the lower measurement.

7. Overbite

This is the amount by which the upper incisors overlap the lower incisors in the vertical dimension. The overbite should be assessed at the level of the centre of the incisal edge of the upper left central incisor. If this tooth is missing or instanding, assess on the right upper central incisor. If no assessment is possible, the recorder will strike through this part of the form. Assess and record the proportion of the crowns of the lower incisor overlapped by the upper incisor in the following categories:—

Use the upper left central incisor at the mid section of the tooth.

1 — The upper incisor does not overlap the lower incisor.

2 — The upper incisor overlaps the lower incisor by not more than one-third of the clinical crown of the lower incisor.

3 — The upper incisor overlaps the lower incisor by more than one-third of the clinical crown of the lower incisor.

IF IN DOUBT, SCORE LOW.

8. Trapped Lower Lip

If the lower lip rests passively behind the natural upper incisors record as:—

1 — trapped
0 — not trapped

Note: One natural incisor tooth is essential for completion of this section.

IF IN DOUBT, SCORE LOW.

9. Dentures

In this section record all dentures whether worn or not. The dentures, including those full dentures opposed by natural teeth or a partial denture will then be examined and the following recorded for each:

(i) **Dentures**

Partial — 1
Full — 2

167

(ii) **Denture Material**

Metal — Those dentures where the major component of the fitting surface is metal not including those whose only metal component is clasps.

Plastic — Dentures whose major component is plastic.

Lingual bar dentures are recorded as plastic.

(iii) **Denture Type**

Tooth borne — Dentures with bounded saddles and rests.

Tissue borne — Dentures without rests.

Both — Dentures with rests and free-end saddles.

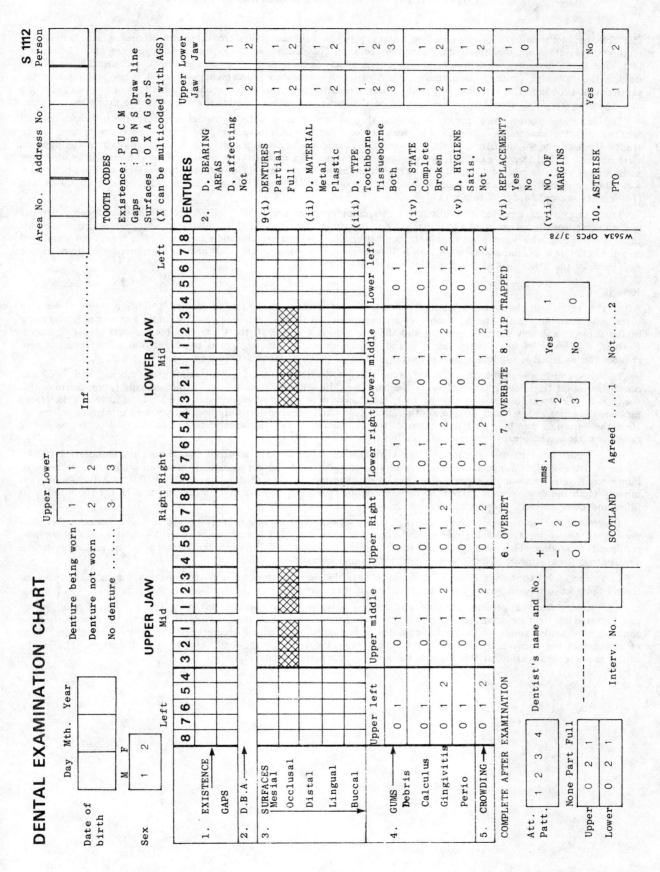

The Calibration and Recalibration Studies

Part of the methodological design of the survey was the calibration and recalibration studies which provided a method of establishing the amount of variation between the dentists in their professional judgements. The studies identified those measures of dental condition about which dentists showed most agreement and those areas where, despite the intensive training programme, the dentists did not show agreement with each other when rating the same dental problem. The recalibration study, completed after the field work, provided a method of assessing changes in diagnostic standards over the 6 week period of the survey by either individual dentists or the group as a whole.

The calibration study took place on the last day of the training week by which time the dentists had become familiar with the examination criteria. Fourteen subjects (volunteer interviewers and staff of SRD) were used in the study. Each of the 14 dentists and their respective recorders was stationed at one of 14 chairs where the subjects were seated. A full dental examination was then completed on each subject according to the criteria used in the main survey. At the end of 6 minutes a buzzer sounded and each subject moved to the next chair. This procedure was then repeated until each subject had been examined by each dentist ie a total of 196 examinations (14 dentists multiplied by 14 subjects).

This exercise was repeated 6 weeks later after completion of the field work. At recalibration the same dentists and subjects were involved as in the initial study. One subject was unavailable and results are therefore presented for those 13 subjects who were present at both the calibration and the recalibration exercises. The time limit employed meant that a few examinations were not fully completed by some dentists. When this occurred the modal score produced by the other dentist for the subject was inserted.

Results

After the results of both exercises had been collected certain measures of dental condition were chosen to investigate examiner variation. A number of characteristics of the subject bear on this study. For example, very few of the subjects had any form of denture and thus no results are present for those variables related to the dentured. Further, low levels of decay were found in the subjects generally which suggests regular dental attendance but also reduces the number of obviously decayed teeth and may affect the scores produced.

Table A shows the results for the variables selected. Variation in judgement relating to missing and filled but otherwise sound teeth was predictably very low and the differences in means between the two calibration sessions also was small. This was not, however, the case for measures of total decayed and filled and decayed teeth (these measures are not independent of one another since filled and decayed teeth are a component of total decayed teeth). Here the variation was high and the means of the calibration for the number of filled and decayed teeth was nearly twice as high as the means observed at recalibration.

Three statistical measures are used in the table: the mean or average score of the dentist, the standard deviation which is a measure of range of judgements in this category and the coefficient of variation which is a measure of inter-dental agreement on this particular area. For example, a coefficient of variation of 0.01 for the number of missing teeth indicates virtual agreement between dentists which a coefficient of variation of 0.78 for the number of filled and decayed teeth shows considerable disagreement between raters.

The results for gum disease also show high levels of examiner variation. Very little debris and periodontitis were present in the subjects and high levels of variation were recorded for these areas at both the calibration and recalibration studies. The mean gingivitis levels showed a major shift between the two studies; at recalibration the dentists recorded a mean score less than half that found initially at calibration.

Low levels of variation and fairly good agreement between calibration and recalibration means were recorded for the number of spaces, overjet and overbite but higher variation was recorded for crowding.

The results for the present exercise are very similar to those obtained in other GB surveys. Certain areas can be rated by dentists accurately (for example the number of missing teeth or the numbers of filled but otherwise sound teeth) whilst some of the more complex judgements show much greater between dentist variability. Thus measurements for decay and for gum disease have been shown to be the least reliable in such surveys. The results in the main results section of this volume have to be interpreted accordingly.

Examiner variability prior to fieldwork (calibration) and after fieldwork (recalibration)

13 SUBJECTS, EXAMINED BY 14 DENTISTS

	Missing Teeth	Filled Otherwise Sound	Filled and Decayed	Total Decayed
CALIBRATION				
Mean*	80.6	182.4	3.9	4.6
Standard deviation	0.5	3.3	3.1	3.2
Coff. of variation†	0.01	0.02	0.78	0.68
RECALIBRATION				
Mean*	80.3	182.1	2.1	2.5
Standard deviation	1.1	4.9	1.9	1.6
Coff. of variation†	0.01	0.03	0.92	0.64

	Debris Score	Calculus Score	Gingivitis Score	Perio Score
CALIBRATION				
Mean*	1.0	5.1	5.3	0.6
Standard deviation	1.7	3.8	4.7	0.9
Coff. of variation†	1.73	0.74	0.88	1.39
RECALIBRATION				
Mean*	1.5	4.3	2.4	0.6
Standard deviation	2.6	3.0	2.0	1.1
Coff. of variation†	1.72	0.70	0.80	1.95

	Number of Spaces	Crowded Segments	Overjet	Overbite
CALIBRATION				
Mean*	17.2	1.8	39.1	30.8
Standard deviation	4.1	1.1	2.3	2.6
Coff. of variation†	0.24	0.61	0.06	0.08
RECALIBRATION				
Mean*	16.3	1.6	41.7	31.5
Standard deviation	2.8	1.4	2.9	3.5
Coff. of variation†	0.17	0.89	0.07	0.11

*Mean per dentist.

†Coefficient of variation = $\dfrac{\text{Standard deviation}}{\text{Mean}}$

Department of Health and Social Services
Dundonald House
Upper Newtownards Road
BELFAST
BT4 3SF

August 1979

To: GENERAL DENTAL PRACTITIONERS

ADULT DENTAL HEALTH SURVEY — NORTHERN IRELAND 1979

The Department is planning a dental health survey of a random sample of the adult population to take place in September and October 1979.

The survey will take place in the homes of selected persons and will comprise an interview followed by a very simple dental examination. Persons who have never visited the dentist as well as regular dental attenders are included.

The survey will be entirely confidential. Only the examinees clinical condition will be recorded and the names of dentists who have provided treatment will not be sought.

A letter has been prepared, signed by me, which will be presented to each person examined. It points out that the examining dentist cannot comment on personal dental problems or treatment needs and that the person's dentist should be consulted on these matters.

This letter is to inform dental practitioners that survey dental examinations may take place in their area during September and October. It is to provide them with information to allay any fears which may be expressed by patients. It is intended also to reassure the dentists.

JOHN R. RHODES
for Chief Dental Officer

Adult Dental Health Survey

I would like to thank you for your co-operation in this enquiry about dental health which is being carried out for the Department of Health and Social Services.

I must point out that the dentist who has examined your teeth cannot comment on your dental health or need for dental treatment, if any. Your own dentist, seeing you in his own surgery is the person to do this.

It could be that you need dental treatment but are not aware of it. Dental trouble, in its early stages, can be hard to recognise. The sooner you know about it, the better for you because it is then easier for you to have it put right.

My advice therefore is that you should make regular visits to a dentist. Experience has shown that most people with teeth of their own, who have not been seen by a dentist for over a year would benefit by his advice.

JOHN R. RHODES
for Chief Dental Officer
Department of Health & Social Services

Printed in Northern Ireland for Her Majesty's Stationery Office
by Nelson & Knox (NI) Ltd Belfast   Dd 622530 K2 4/81 Gp 148